# THE TASTE FOR KNOWLEDGE

*Medical anthropology facing medical realities*

# THE TASTE FOR KNOWLEDGE

*Medical anthropology facing medical realities*

*Edited by*
**Sylvie Fainzang · Hans Einar Hem · Mette Bech Risør**

Aarhus University Press

*The Taste for Knowledge. Medical
anthropology facing medical realities*
© Aarhus University Press and the Authors 2010
Cover design: Jørgen Sparre
Illustration: Doctor examining patient with stethoscope
Book printed on Munken Premium Cream 100g
Typeface: Janson Text and Myriad
Printed by Narayana Press, Denmark
ISBN 978 87 7934 515 7

Aarhus University Press
Langelandsgade 177
DK-8200 Århus N
www.unipress.dk

White Cross Mills
Hightown, Lancaster, LA1 4XS
United Kingdom
www.gazellebookservices.co.uk

PO Box 511
Oakville, CT 06779
USA
www.oxbowbooks.com

Published with the financial support of
Aarhus University Research Foundation

# Contents

# Preface

This book is the result of a reflection conducted on the occasion of an international conference of MAAH (Medical Anthropology At Home), which took place in Denmark in May 2008.

MAAH is a network of medical anthropologists who do research in their own culture and society. The network's aim is to bring together medical anthropologists in order to discuss theoretical, methodological and practical issues in relation to health and culture.

The network was established in 1998 during the first conference of Medical Anthropology at Home, held in Zeist, The Netherlands. The network usually meets every second year to present and discuss recent work. The fifth conference was held in Sandbjerg, Denmark, and covered the theme: 'Medical anthropology, health care systems and the client society. Investigating interactions of practice, power and science'. It was organised by Mette Bech Risør, from the Research Clinic for Functional Disorders at Aarhus University Hospital, Denmark, and Bjarke Paarup from the Department of Anthropology and Ethnography at Aarhus University, Denmark. The project was supported financially by the Aarhus University Research Foundation and the Danish Council for Independent Research. We are very grateful indeed to both of these Foundations for financial support, which made it possible to hold the conference and, not least, to publish this selection of papers in the present volume.

The reflection benefited from fruitful exchanges on a wide range of issues. The articles in the book were carefully gathered after a reviewing process, with the idea of contributing further to what we consider the important issues in medical anthropology today. In this regard, we wish to express our appreciation to the reviewers for their most valuable comments.

We wish to pay tribute to the memory of Els van Dongen, one of the contributing authors to this volume, whom we sadly lost in 2009. Els was an engaged academic and an inspiring colleague in the promotion of medical anthropology. She had prepared a paper for the conference in 2008, but due to her developing cancer was unable to attend. Her paper was read to the participants and is now included in this book.

June 2010
*Sylvie Fainzang · Hans Einar Hem · Mette Bech Risør*

Sylvie Fainzang · Hans Einar Hem · Mette Bech Risør

# Introduction

When the Society for Medical Anthropology in the US celebrated its 50th anniversary in 2009, they focused on medical anthropology at the intersection: '50 years of interdisciplinarity'. The reflection on the way anthropology faces interdisciplinarity and deals with it, is also that which partly motivated this book. But this reflection consists of chapters written – with one exception – from a *European* perspective. The situation for medical anthropology in most European countries is quite different from the US, where MA is the largest sub-field of anthropology. But the challenges are much the same. Medical anthropology is by default encountering other sciences, with other epistemologies, and that creates friction[1] – and friction creates energy and creativity.[2] The encounters with medicine: the medical systems, medical research and medical doctors are especially at the centre. Several contributions in this book take on the challenge and suggest different strategies.

Medical anthropology traces its roots to European anthropology, years before the Society of Medical Anthropology was founded in the US. Evans-Prichard's book on the Azande from 1937 (Evans-Pritchard 1937) and Ernesto De Martino's book on the healing ritual of the tarantella in South-Italy from 1958 (Martinoa and Zinn 2005 (1958) are two outstanding examples. This book shows that European medical anthropology is still in the making and that medical anthropology is becoming increasingly important in the fields of medical research and public health.

## This book

We have organized the contributions in this book into two main sections; the first is focusing on medical anthropology as an academic field in relation to other sciences in practical interdisciplinary work. The other section is looking at the situation in society, with new medical realities and with changing medical systems. We look at how patients manoeuvre in this changing landscape.

If we should look for a common denominator, we could say that *strategy* is one: In the first part of the book strategies for medical anthropologists are discussed, while in the second part it is the strategies that patients adopt.

This collection of papers from (mostly) European medical anthropologists emanates from a network called Medical Anthropology at Home. This network has been organising biannual conferences since the 1990s, when doing anthropology at home became more the norm than the exception. The network has been predominantly European, and included both Northern Europe (UK, Netherlands, Germany, Scandinavia) and Latin Europe, with a strong representation from Italy, Spain and France. We do not claim in any way that this book gives a representative picture of medical anthropology in these countries, but it is still interesting to see if there are trends to be seen from the book.

Medical anthropology as it presents itself here is predominantly *social*. Although medical realities could have been approached with a more culturally or even discursive programme this is not the case here. The work presented is based on the analyses of social action, within the context of health systems. It points to medical anthropology's growing engagement and cooperation with local medical institutions and medical research units as not only isolated approaches to research of health and illness, but as one dimension of interconnected social and scientific processes. These processes are made up by three powerful but also interdependent actors – medical anthropology, the healthcare system and the client society – that influence each other and presumably exhibit a shift of balances compared with former years of medical anthropological research.

## Part I: Medical anthropology as a collaborating science

### Power relations

Medical anthropology as we practice it in Europe is changing, and this is very natural since the world around us is also changing. But what is happening? What happens to Medical anthropology and one's position as a researcher in this collaboration? What happens to representation and intention when biomedicine, international health or medical sociology wants you? Former discussions on this have been held in the Anglo-Saxon world for example, but for now we would like to move on to discuss theoretical and methodological developments based on collaboration. For example one experience for medical anthropologists lies at the level of distinction, i.e. the sharpening of the arguments, methodology and goal of particular anthropological projects. To what extent is, or should, the research process be guided pragmatically by being 'at home' or by strict methodological differences – whatever they are? What are the theoretical implications for a final analysis? At another level we find transformation and adjustment of anthropological approaches to health problems, formulated by and large by biomedicine or other medical fields. Mixed methodology is a challenging approach in this field but is often a tool-based methodological approach instead of an epistemological approach. What happens to the contextualization and critical scientific approach, when it is often left aside to give space to the demand for applicability? What happens to representation of anthropological knowledge? Are new kinds of valid knowledge being developed and/or new standards for qualitative research?

In the first part of this book we have collected seven contributions that discuss this change, each with their own approach. They can be seen as comments to concrete challenges, or strategies for dealing with them. But they can also be read as meta-reflections on being a medical anthropologist in the first decade of the twenty-first century.

Several chapters touch directly or indirectly on the power relations between medicine and anthropology, and between the medical researcher and the anthropologist. In the philosophical institutes working on the theory of science, the battle over the difference between social sciences and natural sciences may have died out. But in the practical field of research and development within health and medicine, it is alive and well. One reason is of course that medical research is a hybrid of natural science and humanities, but it is not always aware of it. Neither makes collaboration easy, and the power that medicine tends to have in interdisciplinary arenas complicates the matter even more.

None of the chapters refer to Foucault and his approach to power and knowledge directly, but the hegemony of natural science, and that part of medicine, is a strong sub-text. But instead of Foucault's distance and disengagement in the description of power relations, these are reports directly from the battleground. That is probably one reason why the descriptions are concrete and practical. The two first chapters go directly to the meeting between medical and anthropological research.

**Joseph Comelles** (ch. I) is trained both as a medical doctor and as an anthropologist. While he writes about 'we' and 'us', sometimes referring to medical doctors, and sometimes referring to anthropologists, in his chapter we read a view from within the medical- or health professional. From that position he sees the need for anthropology, but even though medical professionals can be trained in anthropological theory and analyses, they cannot fill the total need for medical anthropology in the research field. He argues therefore that anthropologists should be supporting-consultants to medical research. His main approach is harmonic, and although he is not blind to the problems he does see good possibilities for cooperation.

**Sylvie Fainzang** (ch. II) takes the opposite position. She sees the medicine-anthropology relation from the anthropologist's perspective, and argues strongly that the goals of the research must be examined, and that we may come to see that the two sciences do not have a common goal at all. Based on two projects, she explains how the medical side put pressure on the anthropologist to comply with its own goal, and that demonstrates the heuristic value of breaking away from such pressures. She argues in favour of anthropologists developing and asserting their own stance, stating that it is by preserving its freedom at both problematical and methodological levels that anthropology has the greatest chance of contributing specific knowledge.

American medical anthropology has played a formative role in the field, and people like Arthur Kleinman and Paul Farmer, both having been trained in medicine and anthropology, may have set the stage for the two sciences working together. They may have underestimated the problems that the differences in epistemological, and even ethical considerations, have brought to the common workplace. Fainzang's call for a more independent role for anthropology resonates several of the contributions.

**Hans Einar Hem** (ch. IV) points to another way for medical anthropology, or rather the anthropology of health. The label 'medical anthropology' is also a result of the assumption that anthropology should be a supportive science to medicine. But clinical medicine is not the only field to research health. The general health condition of a population is only determined by approximately 10 % of the medical system. Other determinants are much more important. This is why WHO in the 1980s introduced health promotion as a separate field of work within both politics and research.

Health promotion is a more open field, without the dominance of one science, and should therefore be a much easier place for anthropologists to work. But anthropologists have shown little interest for the health promotion. Hem argues that medical anthropology has a lot to contribute, and by doing so will also open up new opportunities for work and research funds.

**Sjaak van der Geest** (ch. VI) examines the reason why patients generally do not play an active role in research, and why medical anthropologists themselves have hardly played a role in the development of their involvement in anthropological studies, while he thinks that the personal involvement of patients in research about themselves fits well into the anthropological philosophy in its various phases and with its various characteristics (participant observation, emic perspective, etc.). For him, in the 'partnership' between anthropologists and patients, there is a meeting between two subjectivities.

**Rikke Sand Andersen** (ch. III) discusses the difference in standpoint between the above-mentioned medicine, anthropology and the patient in the empirical case of patient delay. She shows that the medical question of why patients with life threatening symptoms delay contacting their doctor (which is a very relevant question for medicine), is not relevant when viewed from the perspective of the patients. She shows that this notion is connected to universal medical norms, and that the way patients understand their symptoms is combined with other norms, namely social norms. This leads her to address the issue of bio-power, both to discuss the normative stance of patient delay, and to question whether concerns of biological health should supersede other aspects of life. In general, she shows how different epistemological assumptions create different kinds of knowledge, stressing that it is because of anthropology's traditional concern for contexts and its engagement in the empirical studying of meaning and values underlying health related practices, that its input is vital to healthcare initiatives. However, from her standpoint she feels that the research cannot make a difference for curative strategies.

**Sylvie Fortin** (ch. VII) examines the problems and issues at stake that are raised by the practice of anthropology in a clinical setting. She proposes a reflection on the limits and the complexities of the interdisciplinarity, which she finds possible, provided that we consider the double contribution of medical anthropology: applied and fundamental. Those issues are discussed from her experience as an anthropologist and as a member of a paediatric department in a hospital. She underlines the danger of assimilating medical anthropology only as a qualitative method complementary to biomedical research, stressing the difference between working *with*, *on* and *for* the medical field.

*Research strategies*

**Anne-Lise Middelthon** and colleagues (ch. V) have contributed a chapter that stands out both in style and in content. At one level this is a cultural analyse of *fat* and the discourse related to it. But the investigation takes the shape of a dialog between three voices (those of a social anthropologist, a medical doctor with special interest in physiology and biochemistry, and a medical doctor with background in general practice and international health), in order to explore the subject from various disciplinary perspectives. The very structure of the paper reflects their process of inquiry in the sense that it offers separate accounts as well as jointly conducted discussions.

In this way Middelthon and colleagues actually *show a way* for medicine and anthropology to work together, and even – in some detail – *how* to work together. But it also illustrates the necessity of being open to other perspectives and to have the ability to work on an equal basis. That may be harder in a clinical setting than in a pure research environment.

## Part II: Medical realities and patient strategies

### Patient strategies and the structure of healthcare systems

While the first part of the book looks at the field of medical anthropology and the anthropologists, the second part changes focus to the object; first and foremost the patients, or rather the agents: those living with illness, and within the healthcare systems. The contributors have, as their main concern, taken the expressions of recent developments in health systems in a European context. The emphasis is on lifestyle diseases and chronic illness; biomedicine's organisational approaches towards management of lifestyle diseases; the incorporation of new health solutions like complementary medicine; new diagnostic techniques; biomedicine's approach towards dying; and much more. All these dimensions are reflected in both the healthcare system at a structural level and in the strategies and the practices of present or forthcoming patients.

Patient strategies come to the fore in, for example, **Risør's** (ch. VIII) attempt to question and discuss the concept of 'health-seeking behaviour'. This is a concept used very much in the medical domain and closely connected to patient strategies. She explores its applicability through the case of patients with medically unexplained symptoms (MUS). What she finds is a focus on activities and practices concerning health that take place in everyday contexts. This is a poorly investigated area but one of increasing interest for research exactly because the category of patients with MUS, who do not belong to clear cut biomedical or psychiatric subspecialties, challenge the concept of what a patient is and what healing processes consist of and belong to.

The papers by **Meñaca** (ch. X) and **Johannessen** (ch. IX) deal more explicitly with *how* the different sectors of a health system are being utilized by patients, and try also to understand the *hows* and *whys*. Menaca manages to deconstruct a simplified view on migrants from Ecuador to Spain and their use of health resources. Instead of confirming a notion of medical pluralism as loaded with traditional indigenous medicine for migrants, she shows that biomedicine is the hegemonic medical model in both healthcare systems. Both Ecuadorian and Spanish people share the core principles and concepts of biomedicine, but Ecuadorian patients access and approach health professionals in other ways than Spanish patients do, because they are determined by other organising social principles. These principles result in, for example, buying medicine from Ecuador or visiting doctors when going to Ecuador.

The organisation of healthcare, the availability of medicine and the access to medicine is also a main structural factor of concern in Johannessen's research. She compares the use of complementary medicine among Danes and Italians (where her material is collected in the Tuscany region) showing that the very structural organisation and incorporation of complementary medicine in health system and society reveals a difference in the use of it, the attitude towards it and the final embodiment of expectations and experience with it. As such the strategies of patients are in all three examples shown to be inherently connected to structural contexts, healthcare organisation, and experiences from concrete clinical encounters.

Health seeking and patient strategies always point to a concern with agency but not just with a focus on individual intentionality or free utilitarian choices. Agency, we argue here, is with the words of Bourdieu expressed in practices that are closely related to objective structures and a production of habitus (Bourdieu 1977). These objective structures have been dealt with by several researchers concerned with illness behaviour or health-seeking behaviour such as Zola 1973, Mechanic 1992, Alonzo 1979, Kleinman 1980, Garro 1998, Karasz and Dempsey 2008, etc. In their works we also see a dominant situational approach, which accounts for different agents and their social relations that give a specific setting for negotiation of illness. This setting determines the actions and words of the involved agents, i.e. depending on power relations, attitude or social position, but not least depending on the power of categorisation. Having classified a patient – in terms of biomedical classification – as a specific kind of patient creates a specific social relation to that patient and a certain definition and construction of him/her. In other words structural and systemic factors function as a determining frame for social practice and individual agency.

The latter is seen, for example, in Johannessen's contribution that also deals with the concept of medical pluralism and multiple medical realities at a structural level. A growing analytic field of object in medical anthropology is exactly the constitution of the health system and the developments within the health system, but also the extent of multiple medical realities as a growing reality both within the biomedical health sector and outside the biomedical domain (Johannessen and Lazar 2005). Seen in this perspective the papers try to answer what kind of medical social practices develop at the level of everyday lived experience; how the interaction between these practices and the official health system is perceived; and, how we can talk about reciprocity between multiple medical and social realities and at what level.

**Bofarull** (ch. XII) also talks about medical pluralism in the sense that she addresses how everyday life in Spain has always been seen as a source of 'informal support' for the chronically ill – a specific kind of medical reality. However, due to social and economic changes and more and more chronically ill people, this kind of support may not be sustainable and should not be taken for granted. Nonetheless, the public health approach is, in this example, determining the field of care for the chronic patient in line, for example, with the Stanford Model (see below), and may as such be seen as an exemplification of how everyday life is converted into a medically defined category.

## Chronic illness

Transversing Bofarull's (ch. XII), **Gracia's** (ch. XI) and Risør's (ch. VIII) articles is the concept of chronic illness. Chronic illness has become the headline of many political and medical agendas in recent years. The health systems have to restructure their organisational formations and adapt to the growing number of chronic patients, i.e. patients with diabetes, multiple sclerosis, functional disorders, chronic heart disease etc. Models of shared care, patient education and self-care, like the cases shown by Bofarull, are tried out and, from the medical side in many countries believed to be a solution to the predicted burden on the economy and the healthcare system.

One of the central challenges for anthropology when dealing with chronic illness is the relationship between lived experience and the agenda of both medical science and health politics. This makes it pertinent to ask what topics are central in medical anthropology when dealing with chronic illness and what kind of development do they represent? How is the concept of the patient as a complex phenomenon constituted in interplay with both science and medical or social intervention? And what associations are ascribed to patients while medicine tries to explain the disease mechanisms of chronic illness? Lifestyle factors assessed as risk behaviour, i.e. smoking, drinking alcohol, unhealthy diet, lack of exercise and risky sexual behaviours, are in medicine commonly presumed to be the main agents causing chronic illness. Logically enough, it seems, the solution or the intervention to prevent or to care for chronic illness must therefore start with (in) the individual agent.

Seen from an anthropological point of view however, chronic illness is a social construction of which the medically defined solutions are explained by more than medical facts and scientific insights; see for example Gracia's contribution on obesity. Solutions are social technologies in so far as they create and define the problems that are believed to be handled by the same solution (Spector and Kitsuse 2001). This means that illness conditions are not problems or suffering *per se* but they require a certain social context and framing to be expressed within what determines the representation of them as problematic. In other words the framing, which in this example is a focus on individual life style factors as basic to health promotion, sets the agenda of intervention like screening for risk factors or patient education. Certain conditions may be thought of as problematic in a specific way and hence requiring the suggested solution that already lies at hand. The possibility of intervention is already inherent in the representation of the problem (Jöhncke et al 2004). Following this reasoning the dominant focus today within medicine and chronic illness is *both* a consequence of the above mentioned development in etiology *and* of treatments. The solutions suggested are to be found inherent in the individual life style – not in societal structures or economics – because the problem is believed to lie within the individual. A refinement of these solutions is seen, for example, in the programme for 'Chronic Disease Self-Management' from Stanford University, which is an intervention model addressing personal involvement and responsibility. Inherent also in this social technology that addresses the problem of chronicity is that it relies on a common understanding of what chronic illness is and what a chronic patient is. However this understanding is not without ambivalences and is often disputed, both within medicine, anthropology and the patient society. For example, real life experiences seem to oppose categorisation and generalisation of phenomena that are extremely complex. At the same time the category of chronic illness and the suggested social technology as a solution to this problem also has social consequences for the main participants. This is, for example, the tendency to collapse various diagnoses into merely chronic illness, the emphasis on the individual's responsibility to contribute with care or coping for oneself, and the use of personal resources in self-care instead of being able to rely on the health system. Also recent new terms may have profound influence on the discussion of what a chronic patient is and how to view such a patient, i.e. terms such as 'healthy chronics', 'resourceful chronics', 'do-it-yourself chronics'. These consequences of 'kind-making' (Hacking 1992) are important aspects of the interplay between health systems, their intervention models and the patient/client society and their lived experiences.

Eventually it may also be argued that the experiences of chronic patients are not well described in medical anthropology. We have not yet even defined what we understand as chronic illness. Instead we rely on a broad understanding – basically found within medicine and health promotion – that sees chronic illness as a long lasting, irreversible illness requiring medical treatment or attention. In this understanding there is a tendency in anthropology to see chronic illness as disorder, deviance and uncertainty that may be brought to order. Following this line certain dimensions of the condition have been dealt with, for instance the studies by Bury (1982) who has argued for seeing chronic illness as 'biographical disruptions', that have severe influence on identity. Also analyses pointing to chaos, deviance, disorder and meaninglessness as important aspects of chronic illness have been developed through illness narratives (Honkasalo 1999, Charmaz 1983/1991, Estroff 1993, Robinson 1990, Williams 1993, Garro 1994, Williams 2000 etc.). These aspects, also the notion of disruption, have been criticized and discussed though, because they seem to buy into a point of view of chronic illness that lies close to an individualised 'social technology'. Some researchers have also pointed to the fact that different contexts for peoples' lives show different ways of talking about, reacting towards and managing a chronic illness – it is not always a disruption and it is not always experienced as chaotic or adding to insecurity. It may also contribute to identity transformation and it may be seen as a 'biographical flow' (Faircloth et al. 2004). Another recent study, in which the conclusion is close to the contribution by Risør (ch. VIII) in this book, shows that having a chronic disease and 'practicing' it is a delicate interplay between the concept of chronicity and the concept of being human: in other words, trying to be acknowledged as ill takes away the possibility of being seen as an ordinary human being, while being recognised as ordinary, happens at the expense of the acknowledgement of suffering and having special needs (Wind 2008). These endeavours point to the importance of medical anthropology constantly scrutinising illness and disease at an existential level. The concept and the condition challenge medical anthropology as much as they challenge the biomedical society.

Adding to analyses of chronic illness we find a focus on existential matters related to illness and living with illness. **Foley et al.** (ch. XIII) address the illnesses that are incurable – as many chronic illnesses are – and the new models of care with palliation as a core concept that is developing in many hospitals. They show the difficulties in daily practice when attempts are being made to integrate such a model, because it is a new dimension of treatment contradicting the paradigm of curing. Palliation is however an increasing field of interest for different health professionals and health specialties. This may be seen as a result of the growing number of chronically ill and the increase in the aging population, the latter in itself giving rise to new concepts like 'healthy aging'. Palliation taken in a broader sense also covers grief, death, belief and spirituality and such existential matters are becoming more and more integrated into common healthcare, especially within the care of chronically ill.

Existential aspects of severe illness also flow through the paper by **Els van Dongen** (ch.XIV). She tries to tell her own story of having incurable cancer and to highlight the many dimensions of illness with which one becomes involved: for example, the many different medical and social realities that are engaged during the experience of having cancer of the liver. This is both a deeply moving personal story but also a story that addresses important general anthropological knowledge on subjects and objects of analysis.

### Notes

1   See Sarradon-Eck (2008) for the controversy between medicine and anthropology concerning the application of ethical principles during fieldwork.
2   See Perrey and de Thé (2009), where the issue of interdisciplinarity is examined between anthropology and epidemiology.

# Bibliography

Alonzo, A.A. (1979). Everyday illness behavior: a situational approach to health status deviations. *Social Science & Medicine.* 13A: 397-404.

Bourdieu, P. (1980). *The Logic of Practice.* Cambridge: Polity Press.

Bury, M. (1982). Chronic illness as biographical disruption. *Sociology of Healt & Illness* 4/2: 167-182.

Charmaz, K. (1983). Loss of self: a fundamental form of suffering in the chronically ill. *Sociology of Health & Illness* 5: 168-195.

Charmaz, K. (1991). *Good Days, Bad Days. The Self in Chronic Illness and Time,* New Brunswick: Rutgers University Press.

Estroff, S.E. (1993). Identity, Disability, and Schizophrenia: The Problem of Chronicity. In: S. Lindenbaum and M. Lock (eds.), *Knowledge, Power and Practice. The Anthropology of Medicine and Everyday Life.* Berkeley: University of California Press: 247-286.

Evans-Pritchard, E.E. (1937). *Witchcraft, Oracles and Magic among the Azande.* Oxford: Clarendon.

Faircloth, C.A., Bolstein, C., Rittman, M., Young, M.E., Gubrium, J. (2004). Sudden illness and biographical flow in narratives of stroke recovery. *Sociology of Health & Illness* 26 (2): 242-261.

Garro, L.C. (1994). Chronic Illness and the Construction of Narratives. In: M-J. D. Good, P.E. Brodwin, B. Good, and A. Kleinman (eds.), *Pain as Human Experience.* First Paperback Printing: 100-137.

Garro, L.C. (1998). On the Rationality of Decision-Making Studies: Part 1: Decision Models of Treatment Choice. *Medical Anthropology Quarterly* 12:319-340.

Hacking, I. (1992). World-Making by Kind-Making: Child Abuse for Example. In: M. Douglas and D. Hull (eds.), *How Classification Works: Nelson Goodman among the Social Sciences.* Edinburgh: Edinburgh University Press.

Honkasalo, M.L (1999). What is Chronic is Ambiguity. Encountering Biomedicine with Long-Lasting Pain. *Suomen Antropologi* 4: 75-91.

Johannessen, H. and Lazar I. (2005). *Multiple Medical Realities: Patients and Healers in Biomedical, Alternative, and Traditional Medicine.* Oxford: Berghahn Books.

Jöhncke S., Svendsen M.N. and Whyte, S.R. (2004). Sociale teknologier som antropologisk arbejdsfelt. In: K. Hastrup (ed.), *Viden om Verden. En grundbog i antropologisk analyse.* Copenhagen: Hans Reitzels Forlag.

Karasz, A. and Dempsey, K. (2008). Health seeking for ambiguous symptoms in two cultural groups: a comparative study. *Transcultural Psychiatry* 45:415-438.

Kleinman, A. (1980). *Patients and healers in the context of culture.* Berkeley, CA: University of California Press.

Kleinman, A. (1995). *Writing at the Margin. Discourse Between Anthropology and Medicine.* Berkely: University of California Press.

Martinoa, E. de and D. Zinn. 2005 (1958). *The Land of Remorse: A Study of Southern Italian Tarantism.* London: Free Association Books.

Mechanic, D. (1992). Health and illness behavior and patient-practitioner relationships. *Social Science & Medicine* 34 (12): 1345-1350.

Perrey, C. and de Thé, G. (2009). *Le souple et le dur. Les sciences humaines au secours des sciences biomédicales*. Paris: CNRS Editions.

Robinson, I. (1990). Personal narratives, social careers and medical courses: analysing life trajectories in autobiographies of people with Multiple Sclerosis. *Social Science & Medicine* 30 (11): 1173-1186.

Sarradon-Eck, A. (2008). Médecin et anthropologue, médecin contre anthropologue: dilemmes éthiques pour ethnographes en situation clinique, *Ethnographiques.org*, 17, november 2008 [http://www.ethnographiques.org/2008/Sarradon-Eck.html].

Spector, M. and Kitsuse J. I. (2001). *Constructing Social Problems*. New Brunswick: Transaction Publishers.

Williams, G.H. (1993). Chronic Illness and the Pursuit of Virtue in Everyday Life. In: A. Radley (ed.), *Worlds of Illness. Biographical and Cultural Perspectives on Health and Disease*. London: Routledge: 92-108.

Williams, S. J. (2000). Chronic illness as biographical disruption or biographical disruption as chronic illness? Reflections on a core concept. *Sociology of Health & Illness* 22 (1): 40-67.

Wind, G. (2008). *Stiltiende fortællinger. Livet med kronisk sygdom i et antropologisk perspektiv*. PhD afhandling. Institut for Antropologi, Arkæologi og Lingvistik ved Aarhus Universitet.

Zola, I. K. (1973). Pathways to the doctor – from person to patient. *Social Science & Medicine* 7: 677-689.

# PART I
# Medical anthropology as a collaborating science

Josep M. Comelles

Chapter I.

# Should physicians and psychiatrists also be ethnographers? Toward a future agenda for medical anthropology in Europe[1]

To Els van Dongen
*Doctors cannot limit themselves to waiting for patients*
*to come to them for treatment. Our purpose is to protect life,*
*and in order to do so we need to have an interest in all*
*aspects of people's lives.*
(Maxime Kuczynski-Godard, 1944)

## Medical anthropology in the 21st Century

As medical anthropology has become naturalised as one of the health sciences, its professional agenda has expanded. Thirty years ago, research was almost exclusively applied, but now the discipline also engages in basic research and theoretical production (Comelles and Martínez, 1993). With increased funding it has branched out in occasionally controversial ways and because most of what it produces is of applied value, concerns have been raised about medicalisation of the field as a consequence of excessive dependence on biomedicine (Massé, 2001). Things, however, are not as simple as they seem.

Medical anthropologists now contribute significantly to the undergraduate (B.A., B.Sc.) and postgraduate programmes (M.A.; M.Sc.) of study in both anthropology and the health sciences, as well as PhD programmes.[2] They play a growing role in the training of health professionals and in health promotion. Some have retrained to enter the private sector in the fields of communication, and the production of goods and services.

## Purity and impurity

The development of medical anthropology (Saillant and Genest, 2007) has not, however, resolved our collective confusion and dissatisfaction concerning how the field is related to the health sciences. This is not a new issue. Menéndez (1991) has written about the break-up of anthropology into small pockets of knowledge, many of which seemed to be somewhat removed from the core of the discipline. Kleinman (1995) and Hahn (1995) have called our attention to the problems of being located on 'the margin of medicine and the margin of anthropology', and Diasio (1999), in his analysis of the rise of European medical anthropologies, used the metaphor of *impure science* to characterise an ambiguous practice. A few months ago at the AMADES[3] conference in Marseille, which focused on the anthropological training of health professionals, the participants were forthright about their disenchantment with interdisciplinary dialogue, although representatives of the generation born before 1940 – such as Tullio Seppilli and Jean Benoist – took a much more positive view of the progress made.

My own position (Comelles, 2002) is also the result of our difficulties in maintaining a dialogue with anthropology. Our identity within anthropology has also been problematic, and when Massé (2001: 42) writes about methodological rigour and defends our role in creating and defining standard research instruments, he is invoking the devil. For many anthropologists, these instruments are suspect and only fuel the belief that those of us who came to anthropology from nursing, medicine and psychiatry are somehow 'contaminated' (See Wieland and Baer, 1986). Although I no longer hear anybody say, 'this is not anthropology' in debates on the professionalisation of anthropology outside the academy, it seems that anthropologists – at least in Spain – find it difficult to conceive of what such forms of professional practice might look like in contemporary society. What is certain is that, for a very long time, applied work in anthropology – and participatory action research in particular – was looked down upon as 'impure' and out of keeping with the image of a highly academicised anthropology.

If research is subject to controversy, so also is training. At conferences such as those organised by REDAM[4], SIAM,[5] AMADES[6] and MAAH[7], anthropologists tend to complain that biomedicine largely ignores them, while the health professionals present reply that anthropologists make little effort to understand health problems from their point of view because they are too concerned with defending their own professional identity. Two or three decades ago, general anthropologists often regarded medical anthropology with a degree of suspicion that could have a negative impact on the academic careers of medical anthropologists. I am not so sure this is still the case today.

I would not go so far as to agree with Hahn (1995) that by the 21$^{st}$ century all medical anthropologists will be health professionals. I believe that a combination of the 'pure' and the 'impure' is much more valuable, and that, since the publication of the early state-of-the-art review essays by Caudill (1953), Polgar (1962) and Scotch (1963), enormous efforts have been made in research and in the construction and institutionalisation of a scientific community that has transformed medical anthropology into an interlocutor of the health sciences without sacrificing our own professional identity (Comelles, 1984; Comelles and Martinez, 1993, Price, 1992). Today, despite criticism, we have consolidated our position, but we may also have reached the end of an era.

We are at a turning point between two historical cycles. The foundational project of medical anthropology has reached its end partly for generational and ideological reasons, and partly because the wider context of social change, globalisation, medicalisation and economic and cultural policies are no longer the same as the ones that prompted its emergence fifty years ago. The case of Paul Farmer is illustrative. A physician-anthropologist who is currently a leader in the field, he belongs to a younger generation for whom emerging issues define a field of relations quite different from the one that preceded it. This makes me sensitive to the arguments of the sceptics.

The founding fathers of medical anthropology – Foster, Aguirre Beltrán, De Martino, Tullio Seppilli, Gilbert Lewis, Mallart, Zempléni, Fabrega, Kleinman, Menéndez, Good and many others – defined their objectives and research agendas in a specific historical context, before the WHO Alma-Ata conference in 1978.

Decolonisation was still taking place, the medicalisation of the peasantry was in its final stages in many European and Latin American countries, and the hegemony of universal public health systems was in its initial stages in Europe and Canada. In that context the emphasis in the health sector was already on the fight against epidemic and infectious diseases around the world, in the universal development of managed care, in significant changes in medical education and in the recent development of new technologies in diagnosis and treatment. Although 'primary healthcare for all by 2000' was the aim of Alma-Ata, in the West the tendency was to place the hospital at the centre of the production of medical knowledge and education.

From the mid-1950s to the late 1990s, sociologists spoke of sociology (anthropology) *of* medicine and sociology (anthropology) *in* medicine.

Great ethnographers, they understood that in their historical context, the boundary separating the social sciences and the health sciences made it possible to sustain different but complementary objectives. A sociology/anthropology *of* medicine meant that a focus on health and illness could help to resolve issues in anthropological theory *from within* social science. A sociology/anthropology *in* medicine meant being attentive to the questions health professionals were posing, questions they lacked the sophisticated methodological resources – fieldwork based on intensive case studies – to address. Both believed that it was necessary to have interdisciplinary dialogue in which 'the other' framed the problems.

In this context, the split between medicine and anthropology *seemed* to be overcome in Caudill's 'clinical anthropology' and Scotch's 'medical anthropology' –two precedents of the so-called 'clinically applied anthropology' (Chrisman and Maretzki, 1982) – but this was not the case. Academic anthropologists believed that medical anthropology could spearhead the attempt to reclaim a space within medicine without being co-opted by it, or to return medicine to the anthropological fold. We believed, as some physicians did, that the split between medicine and social science in the 20th century should be repaired since medicine – and this is true as well for nursing, primary healthcare and international public health – could not do without anthropology in its margins.

In any case, when Caudill (1953) coined the term *clinical anthropology* he was aware that anthropology could no longer ignore the fact that medicine was becoming increasingly complex and moving in the direction of managed care, a context in which anthropology should make a utilitarian and pragmatic contribution. In fact a sizeable number of services were assessed using ethnographic methodologies,[8] which were also used to analyse the 'two lines of authority' split between doctors and administrators in the hospitals characteristic of managed care. Parsons (1984[1959]) used the same methods in his ethnography of the sick role in the American middle class, as did Freidson (1978) as Parsons' critic. Nevertheless, ethnographies evaluating biomedical institutional settings (see Rapoport, 1959 and Fox, 1959) disappeared in the following decades.

Fabrega (1972,1974) and Kleinman (1980) aimed for an object of study that still reflected the difference between the explanatory models of biomedicine and lay people but from the empiricist tradition of North-American culturalism rooted more in the work of Redfield *et al.* (1934) and Ackerknecht (1985) than in that of Rivers (2001 [1924]), who lectured and wrote for medical audiences.[9] However, by now the debates that emerged in the 1970s and 1980s concerning the distinction between 'disease', 'sickness' and 'illness', 'medical systems' and even the 'mindful body' form part of the shared history of medicine and anthropology. Anthropologists retained – or were left – the study of informal health practices in the context of an only partially medicalised medical pluralism. Between 1950 and 1990, medical anthropology developed a powerful framework of concepts and a sophisticated ethnographic toolkit for testing hypotheses at a qualitative level, expanded its involvement in international health research, and developed a significant ethnographically based cultural and social critique of biomedicine and biomedical settings.

In Europe, however, the emphasis was mainly on philosophy and ethics. 'Medical anthropologists' such as Binswanger, von Weiszäcker and Laín Entralgo, argued against the complexity of experimental medicine and noted a trend towards a relation with the patient that was increasingly contractual, bureaucratised and individualised (Comelles, 1997).[10] As Seppilli (1996) and Menéndez (1981, 2002) pointed out several decades ago, some Latin American and southern European countries developed a medical anthropology at home, initially influenced by medical folklore (see Comelles, 1996; Charuty, 1997; Diasio, 1999), and later by De Martino (1985 [1948], 1994 [1961]) and Gramscian Marxism. Both trends arose out of the contradictions of the process through which the European and the Latin American peasantries were medicalised in the 19th and 20th centuries, and its articulation with capitalism (see Seppilli, 1983; Comelles, 2002). From an historical perspective, medical anthropology emerged in France, the Netherlands and Great Britain partly from the study of indigenous medical systems (Diasio, 1999), though Fainzang (1989) laid the foundations for an anthropology at home in France in a modern and urban setting,[11] and in Italy and Spain from an anthropology at home.[12] Medical anthropology at home only first became a field of study in Europe in its own right at the end of the 20th century. However, its role in Europe is less significant than it is in America.[13]

## Divergences and convergences

Although the discipline should long ago have gotten beyond the debate over anthropology *of* medicine vs. anthropology *in* medicine – a duality developed by medical sociologists in the fifties and present in medical anthropology – the debate is still going on between researchers working in fields of international research and those in the academic or scholarly fields. The tensions that continue to be evident in interdisciplinary dialogue are indicators of the ongoing need to establish and defend positions of power. The reason for this state of affairs may be the double 'impurity' and subaltern condition of medical anthropology, both within anthropology and in those fields of medical practice that most need it: those that draw closer to us the more they distance themselves from the hegemonic practices of 'managed care'.

The less we rely on the hegemonic models of both anthropology and medicine, the easier it is to find common ground, but we are the more impure and the less powerful of the two disciplines. Kleinman's 'margin of the margin' implies that the research questions that constitute this common ground are necessarily also subordinate questions removed from hegemonic interests and the gold standard of scientific knowledge production. The knowledge produced from the shared subaltern position of anthropology and the marginal fields of medicine remains largely unknown in mainstream biomedicine.

The much-missed Roger Bastide (1973 [1970]) said that without self-criticism, interdisciplinary dialogue was not possible. Anthropology's dialogue with medicine – and to a lesser extent with nursing, which suffers from its own tensions – is complex because there is little symmetry between intervention professions and a discipline such as anthropology whose intervention profile is far from clear. This asymmetry is a historical product resulting from the divergent paths of the two disciplines at the beginning of the 20th century. Before that point, medicine shared clinical knowledge and had access to the holistic contextual knowledge that remains the hallmark of anthropology (see Comelles and Martinez, 1993).

So far this century, both disciplines and their respective professions have created epistemologies that reinforce their respective identities and very different scientific validation strategies (Martínez, 2008). Wholesale acceptance of the biological paradigm has furnished experimental medicine with sophisticated validation instruments that tend to be adopted also by those disciplines that share clinical methodologies – psychology and psychiatry, and other professions that, for historical or circumstantial reasons, have individualised their object of study. This is the case especially for those that, like psychology and psychiatry, are prepared to accept the biological paradigm in order to shelter under the umbrella of its model of data validation.

For the hegemonic medical model, the function of present-day medicine is to focus on individual diagnosis and treatment. This works reasonably well in an environment of individual somatic and 'somatisable' diseases. *Reasonably well*, does not mean, however, that it works perfectly, and this is where we find the paradox of the current phase of the medicalisation process, which subverts two fundamental notions: first, the very notion of disease, since a disease category can be constructed on the basis of a single symptom and a technological and pharmacological response prescribed; and second, the very notion of medical practice as the public management of collective health is converted into the individual management of private health reduced to the same disease paradigm. This process represents a complete break from several of the fundamental concepts of medical anthropology: 'disease', 'illness' and 'sickness'; 'folk medicine' and 'survival'; or the 'medical system' as an analytic construct. In the new economic and cultural context, medicine might not have the same hegemonic position it had. It also moves the problem away from the traditional focus on professionals and institutions to a much more complex multicultural terrain in which political economy, mass-mediated cultural production, political models and business strategies are increasingly articulated in local contexts.

It should be no surprise that the current perplexity of the subaltern sectors of medical practice is matched by that of medical anthropologists. For academic anthropologists engaged in basic research or theory production, problems of interdisciplinary dialogue are not framed by these topics, just as they are not in the case of university-hospital physicians who have neuroscience institutes at their disposal and who are often in a position to be able to ignore what is happening around them since the rules of the game of research funding are often in their favour.

In other contexts, the problem is of a different nature. Both health professionals and anthropologists are experiencing radical change. Their training is dominated by the interests of the previous intellectual generation and is out of keeping with their practice, which is becoming increasingly remote from training because it is immersed in the complex tensions between the local and global that are characteristic of current society. The problem lies in those situations in which the health sector lacks responses to local, qualitative issues, and requires technology to handle them because it has sacrificed the management of experience to the management of experimentation. In these cases, anthropology can provide only partial answers. On most occasions, in order to provide a response that is acceptable within the terms of the hegemonic medical model, anthropologists opt to recoup from the market those contributions that have been cleansed of their anthropological 'impurity' and adopt the dominant language: 'grounded theory' for simple field ethnography; 'focus groups' to avoid the entanglements of participant observation; or 'in-depth' interviews based on research designs for clinical trials in order to permit direct comparison of 'qualitative' and 'quantitative' data. The limits of this can be seen in Mahtani (2006), a recent state-of-the-art in international qualitative data production that aims to vindicate the value of qualitative methodologies in the evaluation of healthcare technology. I say vindicate because the author herself is aware that she is attempting to make people understand a value that is questioned by the wilful, conspiratorial or cynical ignorance of dominant groups that are not prepared to relinquish a single slice of the funding pie that they believe to be exclusively theirs.

The problem is not exactly scientific; it derives from a research strategy that focuses on eliminating as far as possible the independence and the creativity of researchers by subjecting the resources that are provided for investigation to ironclad ideological, political and cultural control. Although we now know why no investment is made in the treatment of high-mortality diseases in the third world, we have yet to analyse the non-scientific aspects of current research; that is to say, its political-economic-corporate dimension and the agenda underlying it. Primary-care physicians whose experience or local knowledge prompts them to investigate a particular issue either do so as a personal venture, and therefore with no funding, or they must play the game of producing a type of research that is as 'pure' as possible so that it can pass through the peer reviewer filters, although the final result is blatantly obvious to any trained observer. The problem is that we anthropologists – like almost everybody else in the social and human sciences – have been incapable of subverting this model or demonstrating that a few international publishing conglomerates and a private company that rates these publications have imposed their interests and evaluation criteria, not only on the production of the so-called 'hard' sciences, but also on the others. In research of a qualitative nature that the subaltern sectors of the health sciences share with the social and human sciences and humanities, this is extremely serious, since many of these evaluation procedures can neither index 50 % of the scientific production in these fields – that which is published in the form of articles and book chapters – nor understand that the so-called impact factors in qualitative research would probably record Marx, Weber, Foucault and Durkheim as the most cited writers. What is more, qualitative research affects local issues, where idioms of distress are not easily reducible to Basic English, and any interest that a local intervention or a local problem might have can only be generalised by means of a complex agenda involving political economy and the social sciences or comparative methods requiring considerable theorisation and abstraction.

Some closely related disciplines such as sociology and social psychology have attempted to become hegemonic by inventing new 'scientific' research designs. However, this has meant that they have had to sacrifice their critical sense, their capacity to analyse complexity and contextualise situations, and, above all, the sociological (or anthropological) imagination defended by classical authors that leads to a creativity incompatible with the conservatism of current experimental science, in which the model is still one of clinical trials. These investigations, then, often have highly sophisticated designs but use very superficial 'in-depth' interviews, clinical interviews or focus groups that do not distinguish between information, observation, triangulation and emotional expressions. These investigations lack not only observation, triangulation, but complex documentation: their bibliographic searches rely on Sociological Abstracts or PubMed, but they do not cite books or chapters since searching library catalogues is inconvenient and acquiring the book is even more complicated. The situation is so extreme that young researchers present bibliographies –in Vancouver format, the shortcomings of which would require a separate monograph to analyse – on China, Australia or Japan in English, blissfully unaware that complete specific studies exist on the same subject in the autochthonous literature.

This academic-clinical culture establishes the rules of the game and accepts a common system for evaluating the design, production and communication of specific narratives, research and practice that is based on internal needs but, by virtue of the dominant position of the 'hard' sciences, imposes its culture in order to minimise any loss of control over the enormous funds at its disposal. Because the business of health has only one completely open market – the welfare state sets limits in Europe – it is the economy of the American health sector that imposes its rules not only on the protocols of clinical trials defined by the FDA and subsequently accepted by other agencies – even in Europe – but also on evaluation procedures that can then be generalised on the assumption that they represent 'science' and not something else.

## A new job market

In conclusion I have something to say that is typically left unspoken, at least in the medical anthropology conferences in which I have taken part, but which also arises in discussions of the directives for adapting university curricula to the Bologna process. In discussions on this issue in anthropology and medicine, two principles are excluded. No one in medicine has in mind a curriculum design grounded in anything other than clinical principles – and more specifically on hospital-based clinical principles – even though many medical graduates work in non-clinical environments in industry or commerce in which their medical degree has a certain value. Likewise, in debates on the professionalisation of anthropology, no one suggests that an anthropologist might work in fields unrelated to academic teaching, museums, heritage or applied or basic research. While it is true that Microsoft announced that it had taken on anthropologists to develop Windows Vista, I fear that the vast majority of graduates and postgraduates in anthropology are working in a market that is more and more open, and it is highly probable that their training will often be an important element that determines how they approach their work. This also applies to medical anthropologists. I have not the slightest doubt that our colleagues are ideally qualified to work in business and trade fields connected to the industry of services to the body, in pharmacy and parapharmacy, or in the communications industry. In these contexts, medical anthropologists do not need to have studied medicine. Likewise, health professionals with anthropological training could also find jobs in such markets.

I pose this last question in an attempt to go beyond the limits within which we traditionally move, the limits of a medical anthropology whose main activity is basic and applied research, and teaching health professionals at the post-graduate level. The danger here is that this will be a one-way street; that the health sector will use this training to develop its own agenda in applied qualitative research and in formal academic training without reference to medical anthropology. Our responsibility is to support this sector as consultants in order to ensure that this production will shape the development of basic research, theory and future training. This requires medical anthropology to undertake a complicated exercise of consensus-building since these issues often fall outside the interests of mainstream academic anthropology, and leave the question of the presence of medical anthropology 'within' the health world unresolved. The problem lies in the fact that even if we accept that health professionals who work as clinicians can be trained in medical anthropology or the social sciences, they will have difficulty in keeping up with research advances in this field if they use research designs that remain closely bound to their clinical experience, and we are unable to provide them with an alternative. Perhaps this is what the new medical anthropology agenda, which is yet to be defined, should be focusing on. In this effort, forums such as Medical Anthropology at Home have an important role to play.

## Notes

1 Translation: Susan DiGiacomo, Universitat Rovira i Virgili.

  My thanks to all my colleagues in REDAM (*Spanish Network of Medical Anthropologists*), MAAH (*Medical Anthropology at Home* European network), and particularly to Els van Dongen, Susan DiGiacomo (whose editorial suggestions and careful revision of the translation of this paper have greatly improved its readability), Mari Luz Esteban and Enrique Perdiguero.

2 In Europe there are twenty Masters or PhD programmes at present (Hsu and Montag, 2005).

3 French Association of Medical Anthropologists.

4 Spanish Network of Medical Anthropologists.

5 Italian Society of Medical Anthropologists.

6 The French-speaking network of medical anthropologists.

7 Medical Anthropology at Home European network.

8 See Rapoport's (1959) assessment of Maxwell Jones' concept of the 'therapeutic community'.

9 See Kleinman (2006) about Rivers' twofold identity as anthropologist and psychiatrist.

10 For an ethnographic history of managed care in the 20th century, see Risse's (1999) analysis of its development in North America.

11 The development of European anthropology at home as a network of interests was one of the main works of the late Els van Dongen from 1997.

12 See Prat, Pujadas and Comelles (1980), Comelles (1984, 1996) and Charuty (1997).

13 See Saillant and Genest (2007) for a quite complete state-of-the-art description of the evolution of national medical anthropologies from overseas to homeland.

## Bibliography

Ackerknecht, E.H. (1985). *Medicina y Antropologia Social*. Madrid: Akal.

Bastide, R. (1973 [1970]). Prefacio. In: Devereux, Georges, *Ensayos de Etnopsiquiatría General*. Barcelona: Barral Editores, 9-19.

Caudill, W. (1953). Applied anthropology in medicine. In: Kroeber, A., *Anthropology Today*. Chicago: University of Chicago Press, 771-806.

Charuty, G. (1997). L'invention de la médecine populaire. *Gradhiva* (22) 45-57.

Comelles, J.M., (ed.) (1984). *Antropologia i Salut. Salut i Societat. Seminari 2*. Barcelona: Fundació Caixa de Pensions.

Comelles, J.M. (1996). Da superstizioni a medicina popolare: La transizione da un concetto religioso a un concetto médico. *AM. Rivista Italiana di Antropologia Medica* (1-2): 57-89.

Comelles, J.M. (1997). Paradojas de la antropología médica europea. *Nueva Antropología*, 52-53: 187-214.

Comelles, J.M. (2002). Writing at the margin of the margin: medical anthropology in Southern Europe. *Anthropology & Medicine*, 9 (1): 7-23.

Comelles, J.M. and Martínez-Hernáez, A. (1993). *Enfermedad, cultura y sociedad. Un ensayo sobre las relaciones entre la antropología social y la medicina*. Madrid: Eudema.

Chrisman, N.J. and Maretzki, T.W. (1982). *Clinically Applied Anthropology: Anthropologists in Health Science Settings*. Dordrecht: Reidel.

Diasio, N. (1999). *La science impure. Anthropologie et médecine en France, Grande-Bretagne, Italie, Pays-Bas*. París: Presses Universitaires de France.

Fabrega Jr., H. (1972). Medical anthropology. *Biannual Review of Anthropology*.

Fabrega Jr., H. (1974). *Disease and Social Behavior*. Cambridge: M.I.T. Press.

Fainzang, S. (1989). *Pour une Anthropologie de la Maladie en France*. París: EHESS (Translated: *Of Malady and Misery. An Africanist perspective on European Illness*, 2000, Amsterdam: Het Spinhuis).

Fox, R. (1959). *Experiment Perilous: Physicians and Patients Facing the Unknown*. Glencoe: Free Press.

Freidson, E. (1978 [1970]). *La profesión médica*. Barcelona: Península.

Hahn, R.A. (1995). *Sickness and Healing: An Anthropological Perspective*. New Haven, Cambridge: Yale University Press.

Hsu, E., Montag, D. (2005). *Medical Anthropology in Europe: Teaching and Doctoral Research*. Oxford: Sean Kingston Publishing.

Kleinman, A. (1980). *Patients and Healers in the Context of Culture*. Berkeley: University of California Press.

Kleinman, A. (1995). *Writing at the Margin: Discourse between Anthropology and Medicine*. Berkeley, Ca.: University of California Press.

Kleinman, A. (2006). *What Really Matters: Living a Moral Life amidst Uncertainty and Danger*. New York: Oxford University Press.

Kuczynski-Godard, Maxime (2004 [1944]). La Vida en la Amazonía peruana. Obervaciones de un médico. Lima, Fondo Editorial de la UNMSM.

Mahtani, C.V. (2006). *Metodologia para incorporar los estudios cualitativos en la evaluación de tecnologías sanitarias. Informes estudios e investigación*. Madrid: Ministerio de Sanidad y Consumo.

Martino, E. de. (1985 [1948]). *El Mundo mágico*. México, Direccion de Difusión Cultural.

Martino, E. de. (1994 [1961]). *La terra del rimorso. Contributo a una storia religiosa del sud*. Milan: Il Saggiatore.

Massé, R. (2001). Contributions and challenges of medical anthropology to anthropology. Integration of multiple dimensions of social suffering and medicalization of medical anthropology. In: Dongen, E. and Comelles, J.M. (eds.), *Medical Anthropology and Anthropology*. Perugia: Fondazione Angelo Celli, 41-60.

Menéndez, E.L. (1981). *Poder, estratificación y salud. Análisis de las condiciones sociales y económicas de la enfermedad en Yucatán*. México: La Casa Chata.

Menéndez, E.L. (1991). Definiciones, indefiniciones y pequeños saberes. *Alteridades* 1 (1): 21-33.

Menéndez, E.L. (2002). *La parte negada de la Cultura*. Barcelona: Bellaterra.

Parsons, T. (1984 [1959]). *El sistema social*. Madrid: Alianza Editorial.

Polgar, S. (1962). Health and human behavior: areas of interest common to the social and medical sciences. *Current Anthropology*, 3 (2): 159-205.

Prat, J., Pujadas, J.J., and Comelles, J.M. (1980). Sobre el contexto social del enfermar. In: Kenny, M. and Miguel, J. de (eds.), *La Antropología Médica en España*. Barcelona: Anagrama, 43-68.

Price, L. (1992). A medical anthropologist's ruminations on NIH funding. *Medical Anthropology Quarterly*, 6 (2): 147-148.

Rapoport, R.N. (1959). *Community as doctor*. London: Tavistock Press.

Redfield, R. and Villa-Rojas, A. (1934). *Chancom: a Maya village*. Washington: Carnegie Institution.

Risse, G.B. (1999). *Mending Bodies, Saving Souls*. Oxford, Oxford University Press.

Rivers, W.H.R. (2001 [1924]). *Medicine, Magic and Religion*. London, Routledge.

Saillant, F. and Genest, S. (2007). *Medical Anthropology: Regional Perspectives and Shared Concerns*. Malden, MA: Blackwell.

Scotch, N.A. (1963). Medical anthropology: Introduction. *Biennial Review of Anthropology*.

Seppilli, T. (1983). La medicina popolare in Italia: Avvio ad una nuova fase della ricerca e del dibattito. *La Ricerca Folklorica*, 8: 3-7.

Seppilli, T. (1996). Presentazione. In Cozzi, Donatella and Danielle Nigris, *Gesti di Cura. Elementi di metodologia della ricerca etnografica e di analisi socioantropologica per il nursing*, Oriss, I-XXIII.

Wieland, D. and Baer, H.A. (1986). More thoughts on the fragmentation of medical anthropology. *Medical Anthropology Quarterly*, 17 (4): 99-100.

Sylvie Fainzang

Chapter II.

# Anthropology and biomedicine: a dangerous liaison? Conditions for a partnership

The fundamental question raised by the problem of the future of medical anthropology is that of the role it will play with regard to medicine - a recurrent preoccupation in our discipline (Greenwood et al., 1988; Lock, 2001). When the MAAH (Medical Anthropology At Home) network was set up, I defended the idea that medical anthropology should stick to its own problematics, even though they might differ from those of doctors, with a view to allowing anthropology to play its specific role, and not just to be satisfied as a methodological aid for health questions defined by the medical milieu. I stressed the extent to which we need to think about the content of our conceptual categories and how important it is to free them from the content that medical sciences give them, in order to examine their social significance (Fainzang, 1998).

The point I wish to defend now, takes even further the affirmation that anthropology needs to be independent from medicine. I want to stress what is at stake in a way that is even more crucial given that the partnership between these two disciplines is increasingly accepted and increasingly systematic. The question is becoming even more acute, at a time when anthropological skills are more and more recognised by biomedicine and where biomedicine is calling more and more upon anthropology.

My idea is to begin with the example of recent research on the practice of information within the doctor-patient relationship, in order to show not just why anthropology must not pledge allegiance to biomedicine, but also that the specific contribution of its epistemological stance and of its methodological tools make it possible to renew outstanding questions in the field of healthcare and to give them new direction. I will set out the status of questions as they are formulated by healthcare professionals, and the way in which the latter wait for them to be examined by anthropologists. I will show how, by developing its own epistemological and methodological approach, distinct from the expectations of biomedicine, anthropology can produce different knowledge and results that remain useful to healthcare.

## Developing research in the bio-medical milieu

In France, the medical world is currently involved in a vast debate on the place of patients in the healthcare system. Among the strong points of this debate are the issue of patient information and the questions relating to it: enlightened consent, how a patient is informed of a serious illness and patients' participation in their treatments. It is nowadays accepted that patients must be taken into consideration, must be treated more humanely and that in particular we need to rethink how patients should be informed of their illnesses. In this context, there are debates on the difficulties encountered when trying to achieve this objective: some doctors are sceptical about the competency of patients, others mention their own inability to properly manage the human dimension of patient treatment, either for technical reasons (lack of time, especially when it comes to explaining the medical jargon that they use), or for psychological reasons (the patient's difficulty in accepting to hear about the illness). This debate became even keener with the introduction of the law dated 4th March 2002, known as the 'law on patients' rights', which guarantees patients' access to 'all information relating to their health.'

With regard to this debate, I felt that anthropology must first examine the reality of patient information, without prejudging what creates obstacles, and subject the matter to fieldwork testing. I therefore decided to take up the question of the information passed between doctors and patients, by breaking away from the hypotheses developed by doctors which form the basis for a great deal of research in social sciences and public health on this issue. In such conditions it is up to anthropologists to consider the matter from another angle and to decentre their focus. It is in fact up to anthropologists to think differently, or else their contribution will be reduced to confirming (or not) a question defined by the actors themselves. The required decentring involves an ethnographical study and, above all, the construction of its modalities. This is why I felt that it was necessary to do a double study – patients on the one hand and doctors on the other. This stance initially meant refusing the methodological conditions that I was offered, or even imposed by the medical world, which in particular meant I had to introduce myself to patients as someone working in partnership with the doctors and to report to the doctors on the difficulties that the patients were encountering (I will come back to this later).

The study took place in hospital departments (cancerology and internal medicine) in the south of France, between 2000 and 2005.[1] It covered 80 patients, sixty with cancer and twenty with other pathologies, including chronic inflammatory illnesses or autoimmune illnesses. I met the patients at different stages of illness, some being considered as virtually cured and only coming into hospital for check-ups, some receiving treatments (chemotherapy, radiotherapy or operations) and some under palliative care. They were of different ages (between 30 and 80 years old), of both sexes and from various socioprofessional backgrounds (secretaries, accountants, teachers, medical staff, researcher, maintenance staff, company directors, soldier, shopkeepers, engineers, winegrowers, office staff, sommelier, a sales representative, persons on minimum welfare, administrative executives, service personnel, a petroleum engineer, artists, artisans, labourers, unemployed).

The aim of the research was to highlight the logics and mechanisms at the root of information exchange between doctors and patients: What is the nature of the information given to the patient about his/her illness, and what is the nature of the information that he/she desires? How does this search for information take place within the context of a doctor/patient relationship and how is the information given to the patient? What is the patient's perception of this information and of the way in which it is given within the framework of his/her relations with the doctors? How does the information affect the patient's therapeutic decisions? To what extent do lies affect the doctor/patient relationship and the exchange of information between them? These were the sorts of questions that oriented my research.

Thirty years of experience with fieldwork have convinced me of the necessity of investigating subjects who are the object of an apparent consensus of opinion, as in this case, where healthcare professionals agree that information is now passed on and that patients are enlightened individuals with the capacity to make decisions (for example, giving one's informed consent to proposed treatments).

From a methodological point of view the investigation consisted in observing medical consultations[2] and then separately meeting the doctors and the patients in order to see how the verbal exchange was constructed and to decode the reasons and mechanisms of their acts and words. I also used open interviews with patients to collect narratives on the illness and therapeutic trajectories, paying attention to the context in which the illness appeared, the different stages of its cure-care process, the questions that the patients asked themselves, the questions they did or did not ask the medical personnel, the answers they were given, the conditions under which they were told the diagnosis, the information they were given or not given, and their reactions. There were also non-directive interviews with twelve doctors in order to learn how they see the issue of information and how they perceive patient expectations, with a view to measuring any difference between the hopes that patients declared and the hopes they were perceived to have. When possible, doctors and patients were interviewed just after the consultation. Where this was not possible, they were interviewed later on, sometimes several days later. For some of them, these interviews took the form of a sort of 'debriefing' during which they explained what they had said, why they had said it, what they had not said and why they had not said it. For me it was therefore a case of observing consultations whilst maintaining total neutrality and distance regarding the two parties (in other words, the two protagonists in the relationship). To achieve this, I met the interviewees both at the hospital (in various environments: consultation rooms, daytime hospitalisations, weekly hospitalisations, meetings of healthcare personnel), and outside the hospital – in particular at patients' homes where they found it easier to talk – in order to diversify the places where I was interacting with the interviewees, be they patients, doctors, other healthcare personnel or patients' families. This process allowed me not only to gather data on how doctors give patients information, but also on how patients pass on information to doctors, and sometimes on the lies that each tells the other.

For the medical milieu, working on the question of information means either thinking about how to make a non-traumatic announcement, or making sure that patients have access to an informed consent form that is clearly written, or else ensuring that patients understand the modes of treatment so that they can agree to them and follow them. But anthropologists cannot accept reducing their research to these aspects.

I also decided to break away from the stance taken in most studies that are done on the issue of truth in medicine (in other words, whether or not to tell patients the truth about their state of health), between the writings of doctors talking about their practice and setting out an ethical stance on the question, and the writings of those who speak out on behalf of patients (Joseph-Jeannenay et al., 2002; Bataille, 2003). Indeed, doctors generally see the issue in terms of opinion: they are for or against truth (Geets, 1993; Hoerni, 2004), or in terms of technique: they are in favour of telling the truth in this way or that way (Delaporte, 2001). Unlike works done within the context of these debates, most of which are either texts in the form of justifications for what is generally referred to as 'therapeutic privilege'[3]

(Van den Heever, 2005), or else pleas in favour of patient participation, it became essential to renew the perspective from which such questions are usually approached, without making any moral judgement on the matter and by attempting to decode its social mechanisms. The aim of this study was not to give yet one more opinion on whether or not it is preferable for patients to be told the truth, but to examine the arguments used by the protagonists in doctor/patient relationships to explain their conduct, and, above all, to understand what is concealed and what is implied by their stances and practices on the matter. I therefore tried to pinpoint the cognitive and moral systems in which their stances were anchored, and to assess the conformity of the practices and opinions in order to see how the use, search for, disclosure or retention of information is put into effect.[4]

When I asked the doctors to let me work in their wards, they saw it as an opportunity for a partnership, synonymous with the chance to see whether patients felt themselves to be well informed in that particular ward. In their eyes, the study should involve filling in questionnaires that they wanted to validate and where the question would be asked to patients in order to gather a percentage of 'yes' or 'no' responses. Those who answered 'no' were destined to be considered as being in denial, whilst those who answered 'yes' would be the gratifying proof that the ward was running well. But this is not the role I wanted.

First of all, I didn't wish to let patients believe I was working for the ward in question, something which from the very outset would have distorted the study and restricted the material I wished to gather – a problem that was both ethical and methodological. Nor did I want to give doctors a mirror of their convictions, which would have inevitably led me to formulate questions in their terms, thus preventing myself from maintaining a critical distance from their attitudes. For me, it was not a case of entering into a debate between those who say that patient information is no longer a problem because information is now total, and those who say that it has not been achieved, split in turn between people who deplore the situation and people who justify it; it was a case of revealing the forms and conditions of this information. I therefore had to use other strategies, both at the methodological level (for it was obvious that I would learn nothing from such a questionnaire) and at the problematical level (having no illusion about what this type of 'satisfaction survey' would contribute to social science thinking). Consequently, despite the demand from doctors, I could not allow patients to think that I was part of the medical team; I set up conditions for observing consultations, developing a critical position with regard to the attitudes of the doctors themselves, and, in order to achieve this, to explain to the patients, in the absence of the doctors, exactly what I was doing there and what my objectives were.

In addition, I had to break away from the usual explanations of a psychological nature, used by the majority of doctors to explain why patients consider themselves to be poorly informed. For example, many doctors are alarmed that despite the fact that they have explained everything to patients during prior consultations, the latter complain about being poorly informed; the doctors put these complaints down to denial. Indeed, they systematically evoke patient denial or sideration to explain that patients remember nothing of what has been clearly said to them about their state of health. Under these conditions, they felt the pertinent questions of research to be that of discovering how to fight patient denial, how to ensure that patients retain the information provided, or how to ensure that patients are psychologically prepared to cope with the information provided. It was therefore necessary to renew the perspective from which these issues are usually examined. In this respect, as a counterpoint to the psychological perspective from which existing literature looks at lies, it was a question of 'de-psychologising' the approach to this phenomenon and of examining its social mechanisms.

The ethnographic study allowed me to collect data giving a new direction to the debate (Fainzang, 2006a). In particular, the research allowed me to highlight the existence of information-providing practices, whereby information is not provided to all patients in an identical manner, since it is given in preference to patients belonging to higher social categories, whereas it is more willingly withheld from patients belonging to lower social categories. Observation also reveals that when doctors have no information on a patient's social standing (this not necessarily appearing in the medical file, and the doctor not always knowing the patient concerned), they tend to develop an approximate idea of his/her social category from outward signs such as language, dress, body attitude, etc., all of which are approximate indicators of social or socio-cultural level, so that their behaviour towards patients changes not only in accordance with their social milieu (i.e. not always in accordance with what the patient is), but in accordance with what the doctor thinks the patient to be, after an assessment based on a reading of signs, a mechanism which reproduces if not strengthens social inequality. To the famous social inequality of access to healthcare is thus added a social inequality of access to information, to which a large number of doctors contribute in spite of themselves.

Observation of consultations allowed me to realise that the patients accused of being in denial were precisely those who had been given partial information or information that was not relevant to their questions, which the doctors justified with the patients' supposed inability to understand the real information. We are not challenging psychological analyses – widely taken up and distributed throughout the medical world – but we consider that the issue of information cannot be reduced to mere psychological analysis; we thus propose a different approach, one that is more sensitive to the social context of information: by breaking away from the standard way of problematising the issue of information and the usual explanations of a psychological nature so widespread in the public sphere, the anthropological approach has made it possible to highlight the social mechanisms, and to thus throw new light on the matter.[5]

## Discussion

Of course, a study highlighting problems with information and the practice of telling lies is very useful for the medical world, in as much as lying involves a certain number of risks, in particular, loss of the patient's confidence or 'doctor shopping' (in French: 'nomadisme medical'[6]), and might be prejudicial to the development of a good doctor-patient relationship and to proper treatment. But this is not all: it made it possible to reveal unexpected mechanisms within doctors' conduct which need to be examined if we are to fully understand our healthcare system and the social inequalities it creates. Indeed, the medical profession seems to be, a posteriori, convinced of this utility, as is shown by the very favourable reception that the study received from medical reviews, hospitals and the National Order of doctors in France. Yet through the perspective chosen – far removed from that which the doctors I met might have imagined within the framework of a partnership – my research has made it possible to show what medical practice (with regard to patient information) induces at both therapeutic and social levels.

### What collaborating means ?

In this matter, the debate is not simply that of the difference between the fundamental or applied perspectives of different approaches.[7] The example of the study mentioned above shows that research which does not answer the issues of biomedicine (such as working on techniques for announcing serious illnesses for example) is perfectly capable of contributing useful answers relating to how its conclusions can be applied to the healthcare system. The desire to work in a way that is useful to healthcare in no way contradicts a critical approach to the latter. So the question must no longer be considered in terms of a dichotomy between fundamental research and applied research. However fundamental it may be, research may have a utility that is all the more innovative for not being developed by the actors involved. Anthropology must be able to propose and impose research which, in the eyes of healthcare professionals, has not been thought of and is unthinkable.

The instrumentalisation as such of anthropology is not a problem as long as this does not mean that it is 'directed' (in the way that a craftsman directs his tool). That it can be useful or used for a particular purpose, yes. That it is directed, no. It cannot be biomedicine that defines the questions, or the way an issue is handled. This is not a case of sketching a pejorative portrait of doctors – it is legitimate that they ask different questions than those that anthropologists must ask – but it remains vital, for our discipline, that we do not confuse our respective objectives. Of course, we cannot see doctors in a homogenous manner and some doctors show a clear interest in social issues. Yet even though certain among them show such a degree of openness that they are able to welcome social science research within their departments (which was the case for my research), their questions cannot be identified as those of anthropology.

When considering the changes that have taken place in the nature of fieldwork relationships, Marcus (1997) discusses the relationship of complicity which develops between researcher and informant. He highlights the fact that in the context of modernity, anthropologists might be dealing with people who have a power or a position of a higher level than their own – in contrast with the traditional situation whereby there was an inequality in the balance of power between informants and anthropologists in the latter's favour. This leads him to infer that the notion of complicity (in his opinion a notion that is central to fieldwork) must mean an affinity which places the researcher and the informant on an equal footing. Marcus' use of the term 'complicity' relates to the state of being involved and to the partnership which develops, thus making informants co-authors of the ethnography which is produced.

But equality is not identity, and any equality in the respective positions of the anthropologist and the informant must not be confused with any similarity between their concerns. And indeed, their concerns are not the same. On the contrary, I feel that it is not only appropriate to reaffirm the need to be outside the object under examination ('outsideness is a most powerful factor in understanding', wrote Mikhail M. Bakhtin),[8] actually echoing Levi-Strauss' conviction of the necessity to look at things with a 'view from afar')[9] and the incomparable benefit of this outside position ('we raise new questions for a foreign culture, ones that it did not raise for itself', wrote Bakhtin). But it is also relevant to support the idea that the anthropologist's distance from his/her object must prevail at home (Fainzang, 2000 [1989]) and more particularly when confronted with the medical profession, with whom medical anthropologists are quite naturally led to work. Furthermore, when it is insufficient, this distance must be recreated. Any affinities between the ethnographer and the subject (be they linked to certain options or certain affiliations, be they national, social, religious, political, cultural, professional, etc.) must not be confused with complicity, which I believe, on the contrary, should be excluded, just as distance and otherness must be reconstructed when they are not present from the outset. It is often on this condition that I believe an anthropologist can work effectively. Note that it is because we are not accomplices that I felt it was inconceivable to accept the doctors' request to give them my opinion of any given patient.

Indeed, collaborating means working with someone else, towards a common objective. But is the objective of anthropologists and doctors the same? Is it the purpose of anthropologists to improve the health of individuals? Is it the purpose of doctors to understand the social stakes surrounding illness and surrounding its practical and symbolic management? No. And if by coincidence certain of their objectives do find a meeting point, it is with regard to the improvement of the patients' well-being, for whom medicine and anthropology do have certain affinities[10]. But once again, affinity does not mean identity, and each discipline, with its own identity, must ask distinct questions with its own tools and a specific finality. There is sometimes talk of an 'alliance' between the two disciplines, but the term 'alliance' is also problematic, because it too suggests common interests and raises the same problems as 'complicity'. In this respect, the marked interest shown by an increasing number of doctors for the ethos of the clinical relationship is not a sufficient condition for the creation of a critical stance and therefore for the formulation of research questions of an anthropological type.

There is also the question of the extent to which anthropology can collaborate with medicine. Collaboration is increasingly in demand for strategic purposes: for example, social science knowledge is mobilised by communication campaigns in order to better plan for the reception of messages and improve their effectiveness (Berlivet, 2004). This nevertheless raises ethical and epistemological problems. Not just because, as Schurmans and Charmillot (2007) have shown in the field of prevention campaigns, those in charge of healthcare policies are looking to discover the endogenous knowledge with which to render more effective the distribution of a medical message, the normativity and legitimacy of which are undeniable to their eyes (p. 319)[11] - it not being the role of anthropology to comment on this legitimacy. But also because, if aiding healthcare (prevention or treatment) is one of the benefits that its expertise provides, the vocation of anthropology is not to go so far as to take part in programmes of 'aiding compliance' for example, developed by pharmaceutical laboratories to allow them to ensure a high production flow, nor to play the role of consultant for pharmaceutical laboratories to enable them to establish doctor profiles and to learn how to make them receptive to the messages distributed by the industry and even to prescribe medicines.

Of course, we understand that for purely practical reasons (financial, material, strategic), anthropologists may reply to invitations to tender, resulting from questions that healthcare specialists ask themselves. But this response cannot be given without being aware of the risks involved. Attempting to answer a one-off question asked by biomedicine is to risk reducing the field of reflection by this single answer. By accepting the problematisations proposed by doctors (for example on the issues of compliance or announcement), we risk losing not only the theoretical benefits that our discipline has acquired, but also the means with which to improve knowledge of social phenomena in the field of healthcare.

Haynes et al. (1979) have clearly shown that the issue of compliance, so dear to doctors, can be a problem for social sciences in as much as it is defined as being the extent to which a patient's behaviour coincides with medical opinion. Continuing along the same lines, Conrad (1985) and Trostle (1988) highlighted the epistemological difficulties one encounters when one does not consider the problems which might be concealed beneath questions on compliance in cases where the latter involves examining the issue through a doctor's eyes. Trostle went so far as to consider the notion of 'compliance' as an ideology which establishes and justifies the doctor's authority and criticises the fact that the social sciences which examine this problem adopt the standpoint of healthcare professionals. Indeed, anthropology must be able to examine medicine-related practices, and, for example, attempt to understand the different ways in which prescriptions are used or under what social and cultural conditions these uses differ from those prescribed by the doctor (Fainzang, 2005), without submitting such a study to any biomedical reductionism. But the critical perspective that these authors have developed with regard to compliance could well be applied to many other subjects.

The question is not one of simply knowing how to manage interdisciplinarity, a debate which many authors have joined (for example Janes et al., 1986; Lindenbaum and Lock, 1993; Lock, 2001; Albert et al., 2004; Trostle, 2005; Lingard et al., 2007). Interdisciplinarity raises questions which are different, in particular in relation to the issue of negotiation, even if it too raises a certain number of problems due to the ways of constructing the thinking proper to each discipline, about which Guyot (1990) writes:

> Even though the centre of interest – healthcare – is common to them all, the approaches and problems are not identical. (…) Without doubt, nothing is more epistemologically dangerous in relation to interdisciplinarity than to erase these differences, to conceal the existing gaps between the theoretical presuppositions of each speciality (p. 12).

The question is more one of knowing how to manage a relationship of power, because in these forms of encounters between disciplines, it is often biomedicine which makes the demands and which has the money (as the backer of the research) and which therefore holds the power, even when the research wants to be purely anthropological and not interdisciplinary. The power relationship is expressed in the very definition of the questions and issues, leading anthropologists to work for doctors and answer the questions that the latter are asking themselves. But do they always ask the right questions, from a social science point of view? How can medical anthropology survive this situation without breaking apart?

To talk about the power relationship here does not mean adhering to the formatted 'critical medical anthropology' approach, supported for example by Lindenbaum and Lock (1993) who chose to distance themselves 'from that large group of medical anthropologists who accept biological and biomedical data as an assemblage of incontestable natural facts' (p. x). Even though I agree with Lock (2005) and Scheper-Hughes (2005) in believing that biomedical nosological categories should not be considered as a simple response to biological phenomena (cf. Fainzang, 2000 [1989]), the point developed in this article is not relevant to this debate. Given the divergences between the practical and intellectual perspectives of doctors and anthropologists (Augé, 1986; Fainzang, 1990, 2006b), it is more a question of highlighting the need for medical anthropology to reassert its position in the field of social anthropology. The decision to carry out fieldwork in a medical milieu results from a postulate whereby the way in which healthcare and illness is managed in a society reveals its deep symbolic and social logics, and the relationship with healthcare and illness crystallises fundamental anthropological questions (social distinctions, representations of the body, belief systems, etc.).

Schurmans and Charmillot (2007) used the example of mental illness and AIDS to show how vital it is, given anthropology's infeudation to medical sciences, to place social sciences' contribution upstream of medical disciplines, in order to take into account the contexts of production of the categories of thought and problematics so as to examine their normative foundations and the power stakes. Yet more than giving priority to one or other of these disciplines, I am here arguing in favour of allowing anthropology the opportunity to define its purpose on its own. In a way it is a case of arguing in favour of a right to non-interdisciplinarity, in a space where the work of anthropologists still needs to be authorised by doctors in order for it to be done. It is therefore important to stress the need for anthropologists, when they are accepted into a medical department to carry out their research, to allow themselves to call into question that which doctors take for granted. We have shown this here with regard to the predominance of psychologising analyses within the medical world, the somewhat axiomatic value of which is posited by doctors at the risk of reducing any other analysis to silence. Biomedicine professionals sometimes tend to see no other utility for anthropology than that of providing tools with which to better do their job. For example, as we have seen, the only objective that doctors saw in research on information was that of helping patients to better cope with the announcement of a serious illness. In other cases, and this is relatively classic, they use anthropologists to understand why patients have a poor compliance. Working in the field of health as an anthropologist would appear to be perceived by many doctors as being similar to working undercover, in order to tell doctors what they want to know about their patients, even if their concerns are legitimate.[12]

In order for anthropology to be able to assert itself as a discipline and be a true aid, it must develop a margin of freedom within this collaboration which lets it escape from biomedical formulations of reality. It must assert a different research stance even when it is requested by an institution representing the biomedical system. Of course this is not an easy task, because doctors' presuppositions are so widespread throughout society as a whole that anthropologists themselves, as members of the public, tend to share them and take them on board, just as at the start of this research I shared the idea that the issue of information resided essentially in patients' difficulties in coping with the announcement of their illness. They thus have to distance themselves from their own presuppositions, and, in order to achieve this, to let ethnographic observation do its work, even if this means allowing it to upset their own postulates, often the object of a consensus of common sense in society as a whole. Although not expected by doctors, the problematisation proposed by anthropologists is of a nature to contribute useful results in the field of healthcare precisely because they are defined outside biomedical questions. To assert another form of work, despite what biomedicine expects of anthropology, is maybe the only way of preserving its specificity and utility, unless we consider that the medical perspective can easily be substituted for the anthropological perspective.

Consequently, when we consider the question of whether anthropology is a science undergoing change, we must be careful that this 'change' does not end up meaning 'disappearance', not just for the survival of our discipline but also for the contribution that only it can make, in some aspects, to the field of healthcare. One of the lessons to be learned from this research experience is that anthropology must try to break away from the questions that biomedicine is asking itself. The condition for anthropology's contribution is to fight to impose its own perspective, and to move out of the problematic framework in which others sometimes wish to imprison it. Anthropology must preserve its identity within its relationship with biomedicine, which is sometimes so passionate that it takes the form of a liaison, in order to avoid the latter imperilling the specific knowledge that, as an original discipline, it is able to provide.

## Notes

1   The field of cancer clearly offers a privileged framework within which to examine these questions. The majority of the observations set out in this article occurred within this context, which was chosen not only because of the abundant literature that exists on cancer and which required discussion in order to encourage further thinking, but also because cancer remains a figurehead for 'serious illness', which usually gives rise to the issue of information.

2   In accordance with a methodology which has been used by myself and by numerous other anthropologists for a long time (Vega, 2000; Pouchelle, 2003; Mol, 2003; Sarradon-Eck, 2008).

3   Established expression denoting the power granted to doctors to consciously transgress in all conscience their obligations to patients, particularly the obligation to keep them informed.

4   I did not therefore attempt to support any opinion by demonstrating the positive or negative effect that this truth might have on a patient's morale or health, nor did I try to pass judgment on the situations I studied. Numerous doctors have given their personal views on this matter, views which of course I do not question.

5   It should be noted that the hierarchical relationship, which allows doctors to choose not to correctly inform patients (within the framework of a relationship that remains paternalistic in France), is matched by the fact that patients are afraid of being reprimanded by their doctors, and by the fact (more common among people from lower social categories) that they too tend to hide things from or lie to their doctors. So the study also revealed practices of withholding information from doctors, practices which might also be examined using an anthropological reading grid. In order to analyse them, one would have to consider not only the situation of helplessness and denial in which the patients are, but also the power relationship inherent to the doctor-patient relationship.

6   Referring to the tendency of certain patients to consult several doctors, until they are satisfied with them (be this with regard to treatment, diagnosis or information).

7   Even though it is obvious that a militant position with regard to information cannot be confused with the anthropologist's scientific position (cf. Fainzang, 2009).

8   Cf. *Speech Genres and Other Late Essays*, quoted by Willeman (1994).

9   In French: a "regard éloigné" (cf. Lévi-Strauss, 1983).

10  For MacEwan (1997), where 'the two worlds of medical and social sciences meet (are) especially in areas of preventive care and the organisation of health services' (p. VI).

11  Schurmans and Charmillot (2007) point out that, just like sociology and social psychology, anthropology is essentially perceived by the world of medicine to be a 'knowledge resource' which serves to get around what is formulated in terms of cognitive and socio-cultural obstacles to prevention campaigns and to the provision of therapies (p. 319).

12  Note that whilst my research experience mentioned earlier brings into play specific persons and thus specific individualities, it is not as individualities that they are of interest here, but as representatives of healthcare professions who cannot be identified with anthropologists, representatives of 'professions of society'.

## Bibliography

Albert M., Hodges B., Regehr G., and Lingard L. (2004). *The meeting of two worlds: Social and biomedical sciences in medical education research.* University of Toronto, Department of Psychiatry. Harvey Stancer Research Day.

Augé M. (1986). L'anthropologie de la maladie. *L'Homme,* 26, (1-2): 81-90.

Bataille P. (2003). *Un cancer et la vie. Les malades face à la maladie.* Paris: Balland.

Berlivet L. (2004). Une biopolitique de l'éducation pour la santé. La fabrique des campagnes de prévention. In: Fassin D. and Memmi D. (eds.). *Le gouvernement des corps*. Paris: Éditions de l'EHESS, 37-75.

Conrad P. (1985). The Meaning of Medications: Another Look at Compliance. *Social Science & Medicine*, 20 (1): 29-37.

Delaporte C. (2001). *Dire la vérité au malade*. Paris: Odile Jacob.

Fainzang S. (1990). De l'anthropologie médicale à l'anthropologie de la maladie. In: *Encyclopædia Universalis*: 853-860.

Fainzang S. (1998). Anthropology at Home via Anthropology Abroad: the Problematic Heritage. *Anthropology & Medicine* (theme issue: 'Medical Anthropology at Home: creating distance'), 3: 269-277.

Fainzang S. (2000). *Of Malady and Misery. An Africanist Perspective of Illness in Europe*, Amsterdam: Het Spinhuis Publishers (Coll. Health, Culture & Society), (first published under the title: *Pour une anthropologie de la maladie en France. Un regard africaniste*. Paris: Ed. Ecole des Hautes Etudes en Sciences Sociales, 1989).

Fainzang S. (2005). Religious Attitudes toward Prescriptions, Medicines and Doctors in France. *Culture, Medicine and Psychiatry*, 29 (4): 457-476.

Fainzang S. (2006a). *La relation médecins-malades: information et mensonge*. Paris: Presses Universitaires de France.

Fainzang S. (2006b). Medical Anthropology in France: a Healthy Discipline. In: Saillant F. and Genest S. (eds.), *Medical Anthropology. Regional Perspectives and Shared Concerns*, Malden/Oxford: Blackwell Publishing: 89-102.

Fainzang S. (2009). De la théorie à l'action. In: Van der Geest, S. and M. Tankink. (eds.), *Theory and action. Essays for an anthropologist*. Diemen: Uitgeverij AMB: 36-39.

Geets C. (1993). Vérité et mensonge dans la relation au malade. *Revue d'éthique et de théologie morale*, 184: 56-77.

Greenwood D., Lindenbaum S., Lock M. and Young A. (eds.), (1988). Introduction. (Theme issue: 'Medical anthropology'). *American Ethnologist*, 15 (1): 1-3.

Guyot J.-C. (1990). Une démarche interdisciplinaire dans le champ de la santé. *Sociologie santé*, 2: 5-21.

Haynes R.B., Taylor D. and Sackett D.L. (eds.). (1979). *Compliance in Health Care*. Baltimore: John Hopkins University Press.

Hoerni B. (2005). Vie et déclin du 'mensonge médical'. *Histoire de Sciences Medicales*, 39: 349-58.

Janes C.R., Stall R. and Gifford S.M. (1986). *Anthropology and Epidemiology. Interdisciplinary Approaches to the Study of Health and Disease*. Dordrecht: D. Reidel Publishing.

Joseph-Jeanneney B., Bréchot J.M., Ruszniewski M. (2002). *Autour du malade. La famille, le médecin et le psychologue*. Paris: Odile Jacob.

Lévi-Strauss C. (1983). *Le regard éloigné*. Paris: Plon.

Lindenbaum S. and Lock M. (eds.). (1993). *Knowledge, power, and practice. The Anthropology of medicine and everyday life*. Berkeley: University of California Press.

Lingard L., Schryer C.F., Spafford M. M. and Campbell S. L. (2007). Negotiating the politics of identity in an interdisciplinary research team. *Qualitative Research*, 7, 4: 501-519.

Lock M. (2001). The Tempering of Medical Anthropology: Troubling Natural Categories. *Medical Anthropology Quarterly*, 15, (4): 478-492.

Lock M. (2005). Inventing a new death and making it believable. In: Dongen (van) E. and Fainzang S. (eds.). *Lying and Illness. Power and Performance*. Amsterdam: Het Spinhuis, 12-35.

Marcus G.E. (1997). The Uses of Complicity in the Changing Mise-en-Scène of Anthropological Fieldwork. *Representations*, 59 (Theme issue: "The fate of 'Culture': Geertz and Beyond"): 85-108.

McEwan P.J.M. (1997). Valedictory Editorial. *Social Science & Medicine*, 44, 8: VI.

Mol A.-M. (2003). *The Body multiple: Ontology in Medical Practice*. Durham: Duke University Press.

Pouchelle M.-C. (2003). *L'Hôpital Corps et Ame. Essais d'Anthropologie Hospitalière*. Paris: Seli Arslan.

Sarradon-Eck A. (2008). Médecin et anthropologue, médecin contre anthropologue: dilemmes éthiques pour ethnographes en situation clinique. *Ethnographiques.org*, 17. March 13, 2009. <http://www.ethnographiques.org/2008/Sarradon-Eck.html>

Scheper-Hughes N. (2005). Disease or deception: Munchausen by proxy as a weapon of the weak. In: Dongen (van) E. and Fainzang S. (eds.). *Lying and Illness. Power and Performance*. Amsterdam: Het Spinhuis, 113-138.

Schurmans, M.-N. and Charmillot M. (2007). Les sciences sociales face au paradigme médical: approche critique. *Sociologie santé*, 26: 317-337.

Trostle J.A. (1988). Medical Compliance as an Ideology. *Social Science & Medicine*, 27, (12): 1299-1308.

Trostle J.A. (2005). *Epidemiology and culture*. Cambridge: Cambridge University Press.

Van den Heever P. (2005). Pleading the defence of therapeutic privilege. *South African Medical Journal*, 95, (6): 420-1.

Vega A. (2000). *Une ethnologue à l'hôpital. L'ambiguïté du quotidien infirmier*. Paris: Éditions des Archives contemporaines.

Willeman P. (1994). *Looks and Frictions: Essays in Cultural Studies and Film Theory*. Bloomington: Indiana.

Rikke Sand Andersen

## Chapter III.

# Anthropological perspectives on the biomedically defined problem of 'patient delay'

## Introduction

Anthropological skills are increasingly recognised by biomedicine and more anthropologists are called upon to study what biomedicine defines as socially and behaviourally related issues. As reflected in the 5th MAAH-conference, these invitations often bring along discussions of the means of collaboration and how we should approach research issues formulated within a biomedical epistemology. This is also the case for my research, which is part of an interdisciplinary health services research project aiming at improving various aspects of cancer treatment. The specific purpose of my research is to explore why some people 'delay' presenting health professionals (in Denmark the general practitioner) with potential life-threatening symptoms.

Within biomedicine 'patient delay' in the diagnosis of cancer has been an issue of concern for decades (Antonovsky and Hartman, 1974; Pack and Gallo, 1938). The concept was first introduced in 1938, and defined as 'an interval between the onset of symptoms and the first visit to a physician' (Pack and Gallo, 1938). This definition is also in use today and it illustrates that patient delay studies are framed within the epistemological principles of biomedicine. First of all it signals that patient delay studies depart in what Byron Good has called an empiricist approach to the body, where symptoms are given the status of objects which have an existence independent of and prior to the patient's perception of them (Good and Good, 1981). Moreover, it could be argued that it reflects the way patient delay studies are influenced by a normative assessment grounded in an ideology of health services research; namely that it is both possible and reasonable to make people react early on symptoms. These principles, I will argue, somewhat contradict anthropological perspectives on patient delay, which show that the act of interpreting bodily sensations as genuine symptoms of illness and defining how to respond adequately to these always takes place in a socio-culturally informed context (Good, 1994; Kleinman, 1980; Martinez-Hernáez, 2000). The purpose of this article is thus to discuss the notion of patient delay as it is employed in biomedically orientated research. More specifically, I will show that an anthropological perspective on patient delay raises questions such as to whom and if patient delay is a relevant issue.

## Biomedically informed patient delay studies

From a biomedical perspective the issue of patient delay is of importance as studies indicate that it is possible to improve the prognosis and minimise the need for extensive and aggressive treatment if people are treated for their cancer at early stages (Jensen et al., 2007). Patient delay studies usually estimate that 20 – 25 % of all cancer patients experience symptoms related to their cancer three months or more before seeking professional care (Hansen et al., 2008), and the last decades have offered many research projects aiming at identifying the delayers and exploring reasons for patient delay (Burgess et al., 2000; De et al., 2002; Hansen et al., 2008; Ristvedt and Trinkaus, 2005; Sheikh and Ogden, 1998; Tromp et al., 2004).

The majority of these studies are large surveys which focus on analysing associations between delayed care seeking and different patient characteristics such as socio-demographic factors (Hansen et al., 2008), psychological characteristics such as denial, anxiety or coping strategies (Burgess et al., 2000; Ristvedt and Trinkaus, 2005; Tromp et al., 2004), or the extend of knowledge of cancer related symptoms (Caplan and Helzlsouer, 1992; De et al., 2002; Sheikh and Ogden, 1998). While these studies have provided us with information on the complexity of care seeking, they can, however, be criticised for failing to capture essential features of social life. With a few exceptions large surveys take the individual as the most basic unit of analysis, and leave us with a somewhat static conceptualisation of the relation between symptom recognition and care seeking, neglecting the dynamic and contextual nature of symptom interpretation. This might be a consequence of the methods used. Large surveys often aim at constructing social profiles of 'delayers' vs. 'non-delayers'. Nonetheless, when pointing to an association between socio-demographic variables like gender or educational level and patient delay, the studies can only hypothetically refer to theories such as socialisation, (Cardol et al., 2006) or norms of masculinity

(Mahalik et al., 2007) as explanatory frameworks for their findings. They are not able to shed light on the social context in which e.g. gendered norms or family practices are fashioned and influence symptom interpretation and care seeking.

During the last few years a line of bio-medically informed interview-studies aiming at exploring the social context of patient delay have been conducted (Corner et al., 2006; de Nooijer et al., 2001; Scott, Grunfeld et al., 2006). These otherwise informative studies, however, tend to categorise pre-diagnostic bodily sensations as clinically relevant symptoms. They do not necessarily give us insight into how people initially experienced bodily sensations and struggled with interpreting these as symptoms; often because they depart in the above mentioned empiricist understanding of symptoms. For example, a Dutch study by De Nooijer et al. examines the symptom experiences and care seeking decisions of 23 cancer patients. The analysis presented suggests that the patients delayed care seeking because they were ashamed or embarrassed about their symptoms or attributed these to common ailments. The study therefore concludes by recommending that 'future health education on early detection of cancer should focus on increasing knowledge and providing positive information about early detection of cancer' (de Nooijer et al., 2001). Such an approach risks limiting patient delay studies to merely assessing whether people are competent in recognising a medical reality (Hay, 2008). The studies do not consider the fact that bodily experience and how it relates to knowledge is situated (Garro, 2001). Overall and at risk of simplifying, one could say that patient delay studies incorporate a simplistic, empiricist model of symptom interpretation indicating that people who do not seek medical care act irrationally, or lack knowledge on what kinds of bodily changes to respond to. Such an approach has implications for the allocation of responsibility (it is placed on the individual), and indicates a series of pre-defined solutions (knowledge) towards patient delay that, I will show, real life may not award.

## 'Patient delay' from an anthropological perspective

To further initiate the discussion I will present two cases selected from an interview study I am currently undertaking. From February 2007 until May 2008 I interviewed 30 cancer patients about their symptom interpretation and care seeking decisions. The interviews were carried out in order to learn about the causes of patient delay. Informants were mainly selected based on cancer diagnosis and gender. Prior to the interview I did not have knowledge of whether their decision to seek care had been 'delayed', and informants were never presented to the term 'delay'. They were told that the purpose of the interview was to learn of symptom experiences and care seeking. The cases presented have been selected because they are, in many ways, typical of the stories presented in the interviews and they clearly illustrate some of the problems related to the notion of patient delay, as viewed from the perspective of the patients.

## John

I interviewed John in the autumn of 2007. Two weeks earlier he had been diagnosed with lunge cancer. He is 68 years old, and lives with his wife in the countryside in the vicinity of one of the university cities in Denmark. John is an academic, and was teaching and doing research within physics and the history of sciences until he retired. His wife is a physician, and she worked as a school doctor until regular and invalidating depressions forced her to retire in her early fifties. They have three children together, all grown up and married. During the interview John contrasts his poor childhood in a Danish farming family with the higher cultural and educational status he and his wife have achieved for their family. He seems a proud man, who steadily engages in the obligations and challenges put forward in his life.

According to his recollections the first signs of his lunge cancer appeared in December 2006 where he experienced terrible coughs that would sometimes leave bloodstains in his handkerchief. When asked what he had thought it meant he said: 'Well I did not specifically think of cancer. Perhaps tuberculosis, who knows. But I did think, if it is important there will be more severe symptoms than this.' He did not share the matter with anyone, not even his wife.

Around Easter (March 2007) he coughs blood on a daily basis, which accordingly made him worry: 'But I thought, well, in May my wife and I are going on a vacation, and if I tell her about the symptoms her world will collapse. I knew that I had to be examined, but I did not want to spoil our vacation.' John does not consult his general practitioner until June 2007 and he only tells his wife about coughing blood when his general practitioner decides to initiate further investigations at the hospital.

A series of concerns other than John's physical well being clearly influenced how he experienced his symptoms and how he decided to deal with them.

He did not tell his wife about coughing blood until he estimated that it could no longer be postponed. He knew that she, as a trained physician, would be worried and 'take action immediately', as he put it. Implicit in his story is the concern of a man who for years has taken full responsibility for his family and, in particular, his wife's well being. His wife's world would not only collapse because he had to cancel a vacation, but equally because potential illness was a challenge to the current structure of their life. It was, thus, also John's world that was about to collapse, and he reluctantly had to deal with this. The ambiguity with which he presents his symptoms (as tuberculosis, but not important!) and the fact that he consciously hid it from his wife knowing that she would make him act, illustrates that he himself had difficulties dealing with potential illness. This corresponds with other aspects of the interview that imply that illness to John connotes 'weakness and inactiveness' which contradicts his sense of self as a strong and active man and thus threatened his ability to conform to what he perceives to be stereotypical masculine norms.

## Winnie

I interviewed Winnie in the summer of 2007 one week after she had been diagnosed with colon cancer. Winnie is 65 years old, and she lives with Michael who she has known for 27 years. They live in a house in the suburbs of one of the largest cities in Denmark. Winnie is a schoolteacher, but has for the last 15 years worked as a freelance journalist and publisher. Michael is a city planner, but works freelance as a handyman. They do not have any children of their own, but have taken in foster children and actively engage in taking care of the children of family and friends. They refer to these children as their 'heart-children'. Winnie portraits herself as a strong and giving person. Personal relations are of great importance to her, and keeping up relations takes up much of her time and resources. They have deliberately chosen to work freelance to be flexible and preserve time for 'more important matters than work.'

According to Winnie she can retrospectively 'trace' the signs of her colon cancer back to the beginning of 2006 when continuous bouts of influenza and colds hit her. 'Normally I am never sick, but at that time I just could not recover.' In order to regain her strength she took some vitamins. In the winter of 2006 her stomach begins to 'murmur'. 'I do not know how to explain it, I was just aware of my stomach. You are not supposed to be aware of your stomach' she explained. Asked what she had thought it was, she brings forth two parallel explanations: Several friends and family-members had become sick, and a cousin went into coma and eventually died of leukaemia, and another friend died suddenly of a stomach related illness. 'I thought it was because I was sad and tense. "Calm down", I kept telling myself. I was just trying to make everything run smoothly and care for people. So this – in my stomach – you know, it was a result of self control, because everything was so horrible.' At another point she explains that she thought she might have a defect gall bladder, 'but did not really have time and energy to do anything about it.'

In early spring 2007 Winnie became worried about her failing health. She shares her thoughts with a friend – a pharmacist – who says she probably suffers from an infection in the intestines and should be examined. 'Then, I thought, well, now I am in this "illness-atmosphere" I also have to take care of myself. But, you know, I wanted to be sure. I did not want my physician to think of me as a hypochondriac, middle-aged woman. You know, those who go to see their physicians all the time. But I sat down with my calendar and called him (the physician)'. Winnie consulted her family physician in April 2007.

The distress connected with the illness and death of family members and friends equally established a platform for symptom ('I was tense') interpretation and strengthened Winnie's obligations as care giver in the family and the wider network. According to Winnie, she had to remain the strong part and did not want to become a liability to her surroundings. She did not take action even when considering suffering from a 'gall bladder disease'. Another issue in Winnie's story is that – similar to John – being ill challenged her sense of self. Several times she points out that 'I am never ill' and 'I never take medicines or knock on the door of my physician.' This corresponds with the way she objects to being identified with the stereotype image of a hypochondriac middle-aged woman who constantly consults her family physician, and uses the advice from her friend to establish a legitimate plat-form of action: 'She said I had to go to the physician, well, then I better go'.

## Interpreting bodily sensations

The stories of John and Winnie illustrate that the understandings of and actions toward symptoms are highly flexible and that decisions to seek care are informed by socially established norms, meanings and relationships.

This complies with a number of recent studies on cultural differences in care seeking (Karasz and Dempsey, 2008) and symptom interpretation (Hay, 2008) illustrating that the understanding of bodily sensations happens in a complex interface between a *particular* person's cultural context and illness experience. This means that the act of interpreting bodily sensations as potential symptoms of e.g. cancer is not only a matter of recognition. On the contrary, it could be argued that in many cases only a retrospective perspective allows for a definition of bodily sensations as cancer-related symptoms, because experience and recognition are not *in situ* separable entities. In the cases presented, sensations are equally related to the onset of a number of illnesses (tuberculosis, gall bladder disease) or not related to illness at all (I was tense). Winnie's tiredness and stomach trouble could have been caused by her troublesome situation. Who knows exactly when the symptoms of her colon cancer evolved? And when it would have been 'the right time' for her to consult her physician? Being asked to reflect on when the first signs of her cancer evolved, it could be argued that Winnie is actually asked to respond to sensations as empirical medical objects.

This prompts me to take a biomedical detour. Substantial clinical research has exemplified problems with establishing the diagnostic value of cancer related symptoms and a given cancer disease (Hamilton et al., 2006; Jones et al., 2007). The clinical significance of e.g. rectal bleeding varies within different populations, and the predictive value for colon cancer is 2-3 percent in the general population. This means that rectal bleeding alone is not and indicator of a colorectal cancer and only two or three experiencing rectal bleeding will eventually be diagnosed with cancer.

Thus, symptom interpretation and the act of defining proper action related to care seeking always presupposes a *contextually* informed interpretation; both when proper action is defined in biomedical terms (when is a symptom a predictor of cancer?) and from the perspective of individuals experiencing bodily sensations (when is coughing a symptom). For some cancers, particularly the ones not presenting unambiguous symptoms such as e.g. a lump, this complicates the process of establishing when the delay period was initiated, and it also indicates that the period can only be defined retrospectively. Rather than being a person-bound trait or the result of a knowledge-deficit, delayed care seeking is therefore more likely to be the result of specific bodily sensations coupled with particular circumstances. This obviously complicates the process of identifying when and how to establish proper interventions and it challenges us to ask whether patient delay is always a relevant term when care seeking is viewed from the perspective of the patients.

## Defining proper conduct

The stories of Winnie and John also illustrate that bodily sensations are not only interpreted and acted upon according to their physical manifestations but equally according to their social effects. Both Winnie and John revealed that potential illness was a threat to their lives and their sense of self a breach with normality. By not taking action they retained the status quo and preserved the different tasks and opportunities that constituted their lives. From their perspective 'delaying' was – perhaps – a pragmatic, even rational, response to a perceived life-changing threat. This complies with a line of cancer studies which show that serious illness removes people from their social roles, changes relationships and challenge the definition of the self (Charmaz, 1995; Hunt, 2000). This is not to imply that Winnie and John reflected consciously on the pros and cons of care seeking. The fact that their stories are told retrospectively, probably adds degrees of consciousness and intent to their representations of the care seeking process. Being asked 'to reflect on what happened' naturally brings forth connections and interrelatedness which might not have been there at the time of action (Mattingly, 1998), a tendency that may have been strengthened by the choice of method, as information obtained from interviews is likely to be biased toward normative statements. However, the cases indicate that the understanding of, and acting on, symptoms combine with social norms and expectations and involve aspects of self-preservation that further complicate the process of making sure that people behave 'satisfactorily' in a situation of potential illness.

A line of anthropologists inspired by Foucault's concept of biopower proclaim that people in the modern Western societies are met with increasing expectations to place themselves in the hands of biomedicine (Lupton, 2003; Rabinow, 1996). A tendency that is argued has been strengthened due to the current popularity of testing and screening procedures to diagnose disease in its early stages. Paul Rabinow has presented the concept of 'bio-power' to illustrate the ways that biological nature, as revealed and controlled by science, structure social organisation and individual identities. In line with these ideas the sociologists Rose and Novas (2005) use 'biological citizenship' to call attention to the way that conceptions of citizens are linked to beliefs about biological existence, and where the active biological citizen informs herself, and lives responsibly, adjusting diet and lifestyle so as to maximise health (Rose and Novas, 2005). They describe how such responsible behaviours have routinely been built into public health measures, producing new types of problematic people – 'those who refuse to identify themselves with this responsible community of biological citizens' (Rose and Novas 2005:451). Common to these studies is that they all, through different concepts, describe a process where focus on physical health is enhanced as biomedical discourses provides claims over social territories.

The definition of patient delay as a problem of relevance for biomedicine could also be an example of this. The concept of 'delay' signals a normative stance (that some people need to respond faster to potential cancer symptoms) and patient delay studies are conducted to inform health policies, which, as indicated, have social implications as they equally define problems (what is abnormal; here, delaying care seeking) and their solutions (what is normal; here, consulting the family physician with symptoms as early as possible) (Svendsen and Koch, 2006):

> Health policies are not intrinsically technical and neutral instruments to reach certain goals, they are social phenomena which define and shape notions about what counts as common sense, responsible action and proper ways of being a citizen.
> (Jöncke (2002) quoted in Svendsen and Koch, 2006, p. 53).

One could ask if working with the issue of patient delay is a process of establishing health related norms in the manner of what is defined as responsible action, and where people who do not seek care at an early stage are failing to act according to existing norms and consequently acquire the stigma of being a delayer. Knowing the difficulties of defining 'the right time to act', as discussed above, and the line of social factors influencing decisions to seek care, it should be considered whether we are not risking adding insult to injury when defining these people as delayers? A question might be even more important if we consider the so-called social support-stress-disease theory, which regards disease as a consequence of a complex and multi-causal process in which both social and biological factors intervene (see Martinez-Hernáez, 2000 ch.1). If, as hypothesised by this theory, there is a relation between biological processes and social and psychological factors, isn't it perhaps important to consider other elements than 'the time of symptom recognition' as an indicator of when to consult health professionals with symptoms? Hypothetically, it could have been important for both John and Winnie, that their decision to seek care did not contravene with social norms and obligations, as felt by them. Perhaps some people need 'to be ready' to face illness in order to combat it?

## Concluding remarks

At the risk of caricature, I have examined biomedical approaches to patient delay by contrasting them with an anthropological perspective, indicating that patient delay might not be a relevant issue when viewed from the perspective of the patients. First of all because the act of interpreting bodily sensations as potential symptoms is contextually established. In many cases only a retrospective perspective allows for a definition of bodily sensations as cancer-related symptoms; mainly, as argued, because experience and recognition are not easily separated. From an anthropological perspective knowledge will therefore always be situated and information alone will not 'prevent patient delay'.

Secondly, patient delay might not be a relevant concept from the perspective of the patients because the understanding of, and acting on, symptoms combine with social norms and involve aspects of self-preservation. This led me to touch on the issue of bio-power, both in order to discuss the normative stance of patient delay, but also to question whether concerns of biological health should supersede other aspects of life. What about the social obligations and concerns put forward by Winnie and John? Concerns which obviously complicate the process of making sure that people react 'properly' when experiencing potential illness, and questions the hegemonic status of biological health implicitly stated in the notion of patient delay.

The problems put forward are not placed in order to denigrate the fact that patient delay is a meaningful concept from a biomedical perspective, springing as it does from a concern to initiate treatment as fast and efficient as possible. Rather, my aim has been to exemplify how different epistemological assumptions create different kinds of knowledge and potentially produce different kinds of solutions to health related problems. In line with others, I believe that it is precisely because of anthropology's traditional concern for contexts and our engagement in the empirical study of the meaning and values underlying health related practices, that our input is vital to healthcare initiatives.

# Bibliography

Antonovsky, A. and Hartman, H. (1974). Delay in the detection of cancer: A review of the literature. *Health Education Monographs*, 2, 98-128.

Burgess, C.C., Ramirez, A.J., Smith, P. and Richards, M.A. (2000). Do adverse life events and mood disorders influence delayed presentation of breast cancer? *Journal of Psychosomatic Research*, 48 (2), 171-175.

Caplan, L.S. and Helzlsouer, K.J. (1992). Delay in breast cancer: a review of the literature. *Public Health Review.*, 20 (3-4), 187-214.

Cardol, M., Groenewegen, P.P., Spreeuwenberg, P., Van Dijk, L., van den Bosch, W.J. and De Bakker, D.H. (2006). Why does it run in families? Explaining family similarity in help-seeking behaviour by shared circumstances, socialisation and selection. *Social Science & Medicine*, 63 (4), 920-932.

Charmaz, K. (1995). The body, identity and self. Adapting to impairment. *Sociological Quarterly*, 36 (4), 657-680.

Corner, J., Hopkinson, J. and Roffe, L. (2006). Experience of health changes and reasons for delay in seeking care: A UK study of the months prior to the diagnosis of lung cancer. *Social Science & Medicine*, 62 (6), 1381-1391.

de Nooijer, J., Lechner, L. and de Vries, H. (2001). A qualitative study on detecting cancer symptoms and seeking medical help; an application of Andersen's model of total patient delay. *Patient Education and Counselling*, 42 (2), 145-157.

De, N.J., Lechner, L. and De, V.H. (2002). Early detection of cancer: knowledge and behavior among Dutch adults. *Cancer Detection and Prevention*, 26(5), 362-369.

Garro, L. (2000). Cultural knowledge as resource in illness narratives: remembering through accounts of illness. In: C. Mattingly and L. Garro (eds.), *Narrative and the cultural construction of illness and healing*: University of California Press.

Good, B.J. (1994). Medicine, rationality, and experience. An anthropological perspective. Rochester: Cambridge University Press.

Good, B.J. and Good, M.D. (1981). The meaning of symptoms: a cultural hermeneutic model for clinical practice. In: L. Eisenberg and A. Kleinman (eds.), *The relevance of social science for medicine*. London: D. Reidel Publishing Company.

Hamilton, W., Sharp, D.J., Peters, T.J. and Round, A.P. (2006). Clinical features of prostate cancer before diagnosis: a population-based, case-control study. *British Journal of General Practice*, 56 (531), 756-762.

Hansen, R.P., Olesen, F., Sorensen, H.T., Sokolowski, I. and Sondergaard, J. (2008). Socioeconomic patient characteristics predict delay in cancer diagnosis: a Danish cohort study. *BMC Health Services Research*, 8, 49.

Hay, M.C. (2008). Reading Sensations: Understanding the Process of Distinguishing 'Fine' from 'Sick'. *Transcultural Psychiatry*, 45(2), 198-229.

Hunt, L.M. (2000). Strategic Suffering: Illness Narratives as Social Empowerment among Mexican Cancer Patients. In: C. Mattingly and L.C. Garro (eds.), *Narrative and the Cultural Construction of Illness and Healing*. Berkeley: University of California Press.

Jensen, A.R., Nellemann, H.M. and Overgaard, J. (2007). Tumor progression in waiting time for radiotherapy in head and neck cancer. *Radiotherapy and Oncology*, 84 (1), 5-10.

Jones, R., Latinovic, R., Charlton, J. and Gulliford, M.C. (2007). Alarm symptoms in early diagnosis of cancer in primary care: cohort study using General Practice Research Database. *British Medical Journal*, 334, 1-8.

Karasz, A. and Dempsey, K. (2008). Health seeking for ambiguous symptoms in two cultural groups: a comparative study. *Transcultural Psychiatry*, 45 (3), 415-438.

Kleinman, A. (1980). Patients and healers in the context of culture. Berkeley, CA: University of California Press.

Lupton, D. (2003). Medicine as Culture. Illness, Disease and the Body in Western Societies. London, Thousand Oaks, New Delhi: Sage Publications.

Mahalik, J.R., Burns, S.M. and Syzdek, M. (2007). Masculinity and perceived normative health behaviors as predictors of men's health behaviors. *Social Science & Medicine*, 64 (11), 2201-2209.

Martinez-Hernáez, A. (2000). What's Behind the Symptom? On Psychiatric Observation and Anthropological Understanding. A Harwood Academic Publishers.

Mattingly, C. (1998). In search of the good: Narrative reasoning in clinical practice. *Medical Anthropology Quarterly*, 12 (3), 273-297.

Pack, G.T. and Gallo, J.S. (1938). The culpability for delay in treatment of cancer. *The American Journal of Cancer*, 33, 443-462.

Rabinow, P. (1996). Artificiality and Enlightenment: From Sociobiology to Biosociality. In: P. Rabinow (eds.). *Essays on the Anthropology of Reason*. Princeton: Princeton University Press.

Ristvedt, S.L. and Trinkaus, K.M. (2005). Psychological factors related to delay in consultation for cancer symptoms. *Psychooncology.*, 14 (5), 339-350.

Rose, N. and Novas, C. (2005). Biological Citizenship. In: A. Ong and S.J. Collier (eds.). *Global Assemblages: Technololgy, Politics, and Ethics as Anthropological Problems*. Melden: MA: Blackwell.

Scott, S.E., Grunfeld, E.A., Main, J. and McGurk, M. (2006). Patient delay in oral cancer: a qualitative study of patients' experiences. *Psychooncology*, 15 (6), 474-485.

Sheikh, I. and Ogden, J. (1998). The role of knowledge and beliefs in help seeking behaviour for cancer: a quantitative and qualitative approach. *Patient Education and Counseling*, 35 (1), 35-42.

Svendsen, M.N. and Koch, L. (2006). Genetics and prevention: a policy in the making. *New Genetics and Society*, 25 (1), 51-68.

Tromp, D.M., Brouha, X.D., DeLeeuw, J.R., Hordijk, G.J. and Winnubst, J.A. (2004). Psychological factors and patient delay in patients with head and neck cancer. *European Journal of Cancer*, 40 (10), 1509-1516.

Hans Einar Hem

# Chapter IV.

# Anthropology and Health Promotion

My aim with this paper is to make fellow anthropologists aware of Health Promotion and its potential for anthropologists. Health Promotion is a growing field in research and academic teaching and in the practical field of public health. It grew out of a political will to approach public health from a participatory angle and first materialised at the WHO conference in Ottawa in 1986. The basis for the theory comes primarily from epidemiology, education, psychology and sociology. Over the years other disciplines have also been tapped. But anthropology is indeed very absent in standard textbooks and general publication channels.

There is no coherent 'theory of health promotion'. Two of the most prominent representatives of HP, Kick and Queen, will not even call it an academic field, let alone a discipline. They call it a 'field of action'[1] (McQueen *et al.* 2007). I do think that Health Promotion has a lot to gain from anthropology, but it will require a strong engagement and an active contribution both in theory and in practice.

## Anthropology as an academic discipline

Let me start by a very brief visit to my own path into the discipline. I started my training in what I would call 'the golden age' of social anthropology. The 1970s was a decade when the hegemony and quality of the 1960s had flourished into quantity, when Manchester, London, Paris, Chicago, Boston and Bergen were engaged in debates and discussions, conflicts and disagreements that – and this is the point – comes out of a basic common agreement of what it is all about, the life and work of a *normal* science, as Kuhn probably would have phrased it.

I came to the Institute of Social Anthropology in Bergen after a year of studying sociology in Oslo, and witnessed the first 'wars' between positivists vs. anti-positivists, liberals vs. Marxists. At the Institute of Social Anthropology in Bergen in 1974 there was harmony. Fredrik Barth's theoretical and professional legacy ruled. It was an institute totally loyal to his theoretical position; the faculty – ranging from liberals via social democrats to Marx-ists – all said the same thing: 'learn the craft first, then we can talk'.[2] And the *craft* as they called it, was the anthropology of participatory observation in fieldwork and comparison, in a continuous line from Malinowski to Barth. There were different schools, but *one discipline*.

I do simplify here. Anthropology has had its controversies over positivism and structuralism. My point in calling the 1970s 'the golden age' and take in my own experience is to state something that would take more than a book to argue, but still feels valid. Although I was brought up in the British empiricist tradition, I was taught structuralism, and the arguments against it. Although I learned that French structuralism and American phenomenology were different, it was very much part of the discipline.

To approach Health Promotion with the intention to influence and contribute, we have to clarify what we as anthropologists represent. The problem is that we are *so* out of the golden age of normal science. What is anthropology today? We don't even know what culture is any more.

But I do not despair, on the contrary. To me the historical process of the last 20 years' debate over culture and anthropology is an important part of what we can contribute to new fields like Health Promotion. Personally I have developed, and also to some extent changed, my own position within that debate. The landscape of anthropology has opened up, widened, and given land to many 'tribal' and even personal varieties without losing a common body of concepts and theory, places and history. Last year Ole Høiris and colleagues in Denmark published a book called 'Anthropological masterpieces'. A group of Danish anthropologists, mostly from Aarhus, had picked what to them were formative texts and written about them (Høiris, 2007). I would probably have picked some of the same, and some other texts, but could still enjoy and agree with most of what was written and say 'yes, these are my roots and my source of professional reflection too'.

The common identity makes us strong, but it also to some extent makes us introverts. I wonder if we are a bit afraid of being dominated by bigger and stronger disciplines if we move outside the 'congregation'. Medical anthropologists have made attempts though, some of them being both anthropologists and medical doctors. But the most prominent representa-tive, Arthur Kleinman never seemed happy about it[3]. Speaking to other disciplines has not been easy. Also in the network meetings of the MAAH, (Medical Anthropology at Home), of which this book is a result, the problem of medical anthropology becoming a handmaiden of medicine has often been brought up.[4]

My statement is that while anthropologists have a strong sense of the discipline but lack self-confidence, health promoters have the opposite problem: A strong self-confidence but no sense of *being* a discipline.

## Health Promotion

The field is fairly new. As mentioned above it dates back to the WHO conference in Ottawa in 1986 and the 'Ottawa Charter' (WHO, 1986). But already in 1974 the Canadian minister of Health and Welfare, Marc Lalonde, initiated a report introducing a different view on health, new at least in political terms. It stated that health is determined by much more than biomedical factors. He launched the concept of 'the health field' with four major factors:

- Human biology
- The environment
- Lifestyle
- Healthcare organization

The debate following this report up to the Ottawa conference and the coining of the term 'Health Promotion' was to a large extent political, and WHO was a driving force in this. In many ways it was the politicians coming to the academic world with a problem, not the research telling politics what the problem was.

And the problem was, and still is, that healthcare doesn't work. Although biomedicine has done great things and is developing impressively and with a self-confidence that only some fields of engineering can match, it can't solve the problem, it can't give people *health*. And that was the political insight that became explicit in those years up to 1986; health is about so much more than curing diseases. WHO had, on behalf of a world of United Nations in political consensus formulated the overall goal already in 1948; 'Health is a state of complete physical, mental and social wellbeing, and not merely the absence of disease or infirmity' (WHO, 1948). But the medically based healthcare system could not deliver. Bad health seemed only to increase. It changed character. But as one category of diseases seemed to be tamed, another increased. The pressure on the political system was growing, especially in welfare states where governments seemed to master many other social problems. Biomedicine could clearly not solve the problem. So what could?

Epidemiology was the first helper. Epidemiology is the political system's best helper in establishing patterns of health and disease in entire populations and pointing to possible and probable connections between problems and causes. And that was the first strong insight – it is hard to imagine that it was only 30 years ago – that reached political discourse i.e. that many causes of bad health are in the environment and in the way we live; in lifestyle. So to improve health would be to change life habits.

So what can make people change their life habits? The second helper was a mix of psychology and pedagogy, and later mass communication and marketing. Medicine knew the right answers, so how could people be motivated to adopt them, and how could they most effectively be educated in what was right? Although the political partners here, like WHO, went for the term 'Health Promotion', the academic discipline was from the start just called 'Health Education'.

From its very beginning the field of Health Promotion was rational and *modernistic*, and I will argue that it still is. It seems to believe that it is just a matter of enlightenment. If you smoke, it must be because you don't know the danger. So why not print it on the package; 'smoking is dangerous for your health'? Examples like those really illustrate a very strong trust in human rationality.

It didn't work. And here came the next big helper; sociology. With hindsight, I would link the importance of sociology to some extent to the post-modern turn in the late 1980s and the 1990s. First, sociology helped out by explaining some additional factors, like poverty, social class, ethnicity and gender that form lifestyle and health. But it also contributed to the general reflexivity of society, the 'double hermeneutics' as Anthony Giddens calls it (Giddens, 1990).

Health Promotion still consists of several contradicting positions: A preventive vs. a promotional, a rationalistic, modernist and to a large extent social democratic vs. a more reflexive, post-modern and liberal – or New Labour. What *unites* the field is the normative, and the constructive is the urge to act, to do right. To understand Health Promotion as an academic discipline and a science, the political aspect, the normative view of health and wellbeing, and the link to practical professional work, must be taken into account and – to the extent possible – understood. My take on this is that Health Promotion comes from politics, from moral norms, from doing good – and must be understood as that.

The preventive health part of this is well known and clear. Part of this work has realized the limits of enlightenment and moved to legislation, like the WHO campaigns against tobacco under Gro Harlem Brundtland's leadership. But it still is a huge field of both research and practice going into what works; how can information and education change people's habits and lifestyle? And the quest for evidence-based Health Promotion is alive and well.

The other part, the reflexive and less rationalistic, can be seen as a post-modern reaction to the moralistic lifestyle campaigns. It was obvious already in the 1980s that the preventive approach to lifestyle could easily be taken as blaming the individual: you are responsible for your own health because health is determined by your lifestyle. Consequently the victim of ill health was to be blamed.

A part of Health Promotion, probably the more sociologically oriented part, saw this as an injustice, and focused more, for example, on the macro reasons in social class, and looked for ways to help people take control over their own lives on the micro level. *Empowerment* was an important entry into that. This was taken in two steps manifested in the outcomes of the international conferences held. The conference in Sundsvall in Sweden in 1991 focused on *empowerment* (WHO, 1991). The key elements of 'a democratic health promotion approach' were seen to be empowerment and community participation (Tones and Green, 2004).

The second step was including a *global* perspective and was summed up in Jakarta in 1997 (WHO, 1997). Here the rights-based approach was introduced. Health was seen as both a right and an instrument to social and economic development. It envisaged the 'ultimate goal' of Health Promotion as increasing health expectancy by means of action directed at the determinants of health in order to create the greatest health gain, contribute to the reduction of inequities, further human rights and build social capital. It was also pointing to partnership as a strategy,[5] with civil society or the private sector (Tones and Green, 2004).


## The theoretical and practical approach to Health Promotion

Health Promotion is strange to someone like me, who came into anthropology in the golden age, when we agreed about most things but discussed and disagreed a lot. In Health Promotion I find that we *disagree* fundamentally about a lot of things, but we do not talk about it much. Fundamental epistemological discussions are rare. The answer, I believe, is in the political and normative engagement. We – the health promoters – are 'do-gooders'.

The closest I have come to finding a theory of health promoting empowerment is the Israeli sociologist Anton Antonovsky's theory of salutogenesis (Antonovsky, 1979, 1987, 2000). His theory is directed at stress and coping, and his key concept is a *sense of coherence*. But it actually doesn't relate clearly to empowerment or provide a strategy for empowering people to deal with determinants of health. It has, nevertheless, met a need to operationalize *coping* as an empowerment strategy. And it does make a very important point: health is *not* lack of disease.

The lack of theory in HP triggered two grand old representatives of the field: David McQueen and Ilona Kickbusch, both instrumental in the making of the Ottawa Charter, to create a group of scholars to work on theory in HP. In the book that resulted from the workgroup, they have suggestions, but very tentative ones. And they are very clear on the limited theory development within the field (McQueen *et al.*, 2007).

The practical approaches in Health Promotion are far more developed and seem little hampered by lack of theory. Health Promotion strategies can be divided into three categories according to the group or problem they target:

- Groups with special problems, habits or diseases (tobacco, obesity)
- Population segment (youth, elderly, ethnic minority, women)
- Special settings (community, school, hospital, the workplace, even city)

The first strategy has been the basis for educational campaigns to prevent the development of health problems. The second, targeting special segments of the population, has been a mix of campaigns directed at target groups, and working within settings, directed to one special group in the setting.

To work in a setting has been the main strategy for the empowerment approach to Health Promotion. That can also be divided into two categories; working *in* and working *with* a setting. Working *in* a setting is not so different from the first two approaches, but uses the structured environment of the setting to make the campaign or education more effective. Working *with* a setting is more ambitious. This is about changing the whole setting into a health-promoting environment. Working with a campaign on better nutrition could be done by going into a school and teaching the students. But to make the school a health promoting school would be to work with all aspects of life in the school to make it a totally health promoting place to be, and to make all participants think health promotion. WHO has over the years had some grand programmes for Health Promoting Schools, Health Promoting Hospitals, Health Promoting Workplaces; even Healthy Cities.

## What is in it for us anthropologists?

Not only did I come to anthropology in the golden age, I also experienced the golden age of progressive politics in the late 1960s and early 1970s. And I still believe that science is politics, and that we should look for opportunities to apply our insight and act in society.

As I explained above, Health Promotion is about acting in the world, normatively and constructively. To me to be part of that is important in itself. Anthropology does not have a strong track record in political and practical application of knowledge, although there are some exceptions, some of which are in the field of medical anthropology. But look at one of the most prominent scholars of our field, Paul Farmer: When he wants to do something practical he turns into a medical doctor (Farmer, 1992, 2004, 2005). Or we – at least we feel that we – become the medical profession's assistant and handmaiden if we work together on practical projects.

Health Promotion offers an alternative field where we can be anthropologists in our own right, and be recognized for that – I believe.

Then there is the trivial detail of making a living. Health Promotion is a fast growing field. Thanks to the political side of it, driven by WHO and national agencies, health promoters are in demand, health promotion programmes are in need of manpower, and all are in need of research and scientific insight into the field. And since it is a new field, and still far from a normal science, it is open to new ideas and parallel paradigms. I don't have any statistics but there are quite a lot of universities in Europe and North America that offer post-graduate degrees in Health Promotion (not counting Public Health or Social Medicine). The EU financed a project in 2003 that proposed a standard for a European Master's degree in Health Promotion. We have two universities in Norway that offer such programmes, and I would guess as many as 30-40 in the rest of Europe.

To me the field has offered an opportunity to combine all this. As an associate professor at a university college in Norway I have had the opportunity over the last 15 years to work with research in medical anthropology, development in the practical field of the welfare state and educating master's degree students in Health Promotion.

## What is in it for Health Promotion:
## What can medical anthropology offer?

Here I will limit myself to point to some of the themes where anthropology can contribute with a different perspective.

### What is health?

The obvious question for Health Promotion is of course *what is health*? Textbooks in the field gives several answers, usually starting with the WHO definition from 1948 (WHO, 1948): 'the state of complete physical, mental and social wellbeing'. That helped us move away from a medical definition of health as being 'not sick'. But what does that mean? The originally anthropological differentiation between illness and disease has come to Health Promotion via sociology. Antonovsky (Antonovsky, 2000) and several others (Hanson, 2004) have made the distinction between health and disease, using the concepts of salutogenetic and pathogenetic. But I find that this is still a very undeveloped field. Medical anthropology has a very, very strong and long record of empirical and cultural studies of diseases starting from Rivers' studies of soldiers with mental problems after WW1 (Young, 1995). But what is health, what is the good life, what helps people to build a good life; or rather what do they do to build their life? This has always been a part of the study of cultural values, but Health Promotion requires a focus on the concrete strategies and empirical processes people engage in to cope.

This is actually a challenge to both Health Promotion and anthropology. Over the last years a new field of research on *happiness* has developed. Thomas Hylland Eriksen, professor in social anthropology at the University of Oslo, has started to investigate the field (Eriksen, 2008) in a book about happiness in the Norwegian *over*-affluent society. Affluence as a source of the good life, was also investigated by Marshall Sahlins in his brilliant essay 'The Original Affluent Society' first published in 1968 (Sahlins, 1972). Remarks on *the good life* may occur in monographs. But the more systematic study of health in the meaning of wellbeing, happiness and what constitutes the good life is not a strong part of anthropology. It should be an excellent topic for cross-cultural comparison.

## Comparing health systems

Internationally, Health Promotion looks for comparative studies on health systems. In the curriculum for the European Master's degree in Health Promotion students have to compare the health system in one other European country with the system in their own country.

Anthropology has studied *health systems* since the Azande (Evans-Pritchard, 1937) and Arthur Kleinman has even given us a theoretical framework for it (Kleinman, 1978) that we may or may not adopt. But comparative studies are to me part of the backbone of anthropology, and are studies to which we could easily make extremely important contributions. Today we do have comparative studies of politics and policies in political science and studies of the effectiveness of health services within economics and management studies. But solid, empirical studies of how people experience and use health and welfare services, compared between countries or even between settings are in great demand.

## The welfare state

After the seminal studies of African political systems in British anthropology in the 1940s and '50s and local level politics in the 1960s and '70s, politics went out of fashion for a couple of decades. But the last decade has produced some very interesting new approaches. One of them is the study of the welfare state. One example of this from Norway is Professor Halvard Vike and colleagues at the University of Oslo (Vike, 1996, 1998, 2004; Vike *et al.*, 2002). But the contributions are wider than that, and will probably increase as especially the Nordic welfare states may show more resilience in the time of economic crises than most other systems.

These studies build on two fields of study that have had some attention from a few anthropologists though: the study of *bureaucracy* and the study of the *state* as a political system. The first are studies like Hertzfeldt (Herzfeld, 1992) and Heyman (Heyman, 1995), but also studies in the periphery of the state, like Das (Das and Poole, 2004). The second is an important turn to study the state as a political factor in society as an institution of power with the ability to discipline its subjects and sometimes oppress (Kapferer, 1988; Scott, 1998), but also to protect and provide. This has been evident in failed states in the postcolonial era.

In Europe the state plays a central role in every person's life, and the relation between the citizen and the state is a major factor in everyone's life. The democratic norm and the need for participation in the formation of health and health services is a central part of health policy. But how does it work? Is participation actually an advanced way of disciplining in the Foucault sense, or is it real democracy?

## The ethnography of settings

The three themes mentioned above, the concept of health, the health system and the welfare state, are only a few of many possible themes where not only medical anthropology, but anthropology in general can contribute substantially to Health Promotion. The reason is that anthropology has a tradition of focusing on small-scale society, interaction in groups and local communities. We focus on people's life worlds, how they create meaning. And first and foremost we do that through fieldwork, through participation. This is what I think anthropology really can give to Health Promotion: The hands-on method of studying real people in real life. So many of the studies done in Health Promotion are quantitative, and use constructed concepts and models hatched in ivory towers.

The settings approach in Health Promotion mentioned above is particularly ethnographic in the sense that it involves working with local level groups and communities. To engage in a local setting, the health promoter has to understand some of the things going on there and, to do that, they have to switch between observation and participation, between the outsider and the insider. Just like the ethnographer.

Our master's degree students at Vestfold University College are given the task to do ethnography in the setting that they have chosen to study and write their theses about. They have to look at basic questions:

- Who are the *actors* in the setting?
- What are they doing, their main activity?
- Why do they do it? Their aim and rationale.
- How do they do it? Their organisation and technology.
- Why this way? Local culture, values and meaning.
- What are the conditions? What can they draw on and what limits them in the environment? Infrastructure, language, knowledge.
- What did they do in the past? History and comparison in time.
- What do they do in other places? Comparison with similar settings in other cultures.

In working on ethnographic descriptions of the local setting, the students have to take a step backwards from the setting they usually know well and where they take most things for granted. That helps them question local culture and conditions, and being able to help and assist the members of the setting to put their own questions and empower them to find their own answers.

A debate that may come out of an ethnographic approach to Health Promotion in settings, a debate I will welcome, is the normative and political aspect of ethnographic research. Most of us that were trained as anthropologists before the 1990s got a fair ration of cultural relativism in our baggage, and also a dose of neutrality, or even objectivity in the positivist era. Though the positivist era is long past, the cultural relativism and neutrality will still be there, more or less tacit. I think a debate on these questions in the context of ethnographic approaches to Health Promotion will be very fruitful for all parties.

## Notes

1  But they do try to initiate an entering point, or actually several, to theory building. Anthropologists should take that as an invitation – I think.

2  For Scandinavian speakers see Hem (1999).

3  Ronnie Frankenberg, the father figure in British medical anthropology, told us at a seminar in Oslo back in 1996, that he had written a review of Kleinman's book 'Rethinking Psychiatry'. Frankenberg had given it a very good review. But Kleinman answered him in a letter that it wasn't really any help in that anthropologists like Frankenberg appreciated his book as long as he didn't manage to reach into the medical community. And he obviously didn't feel that he had.

4  See Sylvie Fainzang's chapter in this book for an illustrative example.

5  This was following a trend in development work that started in the 1990s among international NGOs. In many ways Health Promotion as taught and practiced in the West, and Development Studies as taught and practiced in parts of the third world, at least how I know it in East Africa and South Asia, are very closely related.

## Bibliography

Antonovsky, A. (1979). *Health, Stress and Coping*. San Francisco: Jossey-Bass.

Antonovsky, A. (1987). *Unraveling the Mystery of Health. How people manage stress and stay well.* San Francisco: Jossey-Bass.

Antonovsky, A. (2000). *Helbredets mysterium. At tåle stress og forblive rask.* København: Hans Reitzels Forlag.

Das, V. and Poole, D., (eds.) (2004). *Anthropology in the Margins of the State.* Santa Fe: School of American Research Press.

Eriksen, T.H. (2008). *Storeulvsyndromet. Jakten på lykken i overflodssamfunnet.* Oslo: Aschehoug.

Evans-Pritchard, E.E. (1937). *Witchcraft, Oracles and Magic among the Azande.* Oxford: Clarendon.

Farmer, P. (1992). *Aids and Accusation. Haiti and the Geography of Blame.* Berkeley: University of California Press.

Farmer, P. (2004). An Anthropology of Structural Violence. *Current Anthropology* 45(3): 305-326.

Farmer, P. (2005). *Pathologies of Power. Health, Human Rights, and the new War on the Poor.* Berkeley: University of California Press.

Giddens, A. (1990). *The consequences of modernity.* Cambridge: Polity Press.

Hanson, A. (2004). *Hälsopromotion i arbetslivet.* Malmö, Sverige: Studentlitteratur.

Hem, H.-E. (1999). 'Jeg gikk på Bergensskolen': gjenlesning av "Models" i jakten på faglige røtter. Norsk antropologisk tidsskrift 10 (1): 37-52.

Herzfeld, M. (1992). *The Social Production of Indifference. Exploring the Symbolic Roots of Western Bureaucracy.* Chicago: University of Chicago Press.

Heyman, J. McC. (1995). Putting Power in the Anthropology of Bureaucracy. The Imagination Service at the Naturalization Service at the Mexico-United States Border. *Current Anthropology,* 16 (2): 261-287.

Høiris, O., (ed.) (2007). *Antropologiske mesterværker.* Aarhus: Aarhus Universitetsforlag.

Kapferer, B. (1988). *Legends of People. Myths of State. Violence, Intolerance and Political Culture in Sri Lanka and Australia.* Washington: Smithsonian Institustion Press.

Kleinman, A. (1978). Concepts and a model for the comparison of medical systems as cultural systems. *Social Science and Medicine,* 12 (2B): 85-94.

McQueen, D.V., I. Kickbusch, L. Potvin, J.M. Pelikan, L. Balbo and T. Abel, (eds.) (2007). *Health and Modernity. The Role of Theory in Health Promotion.* New York: Springer.

Sahlins, M. (1972). *Stone Age Economics.* London: Tavistock Publications.

Scott, J.C. (1998). *Seeing Like a State. How Certain Schemes to Improve the Human Condition Have Failed.* New Haven and London: Yale University Press.

Tones, K. and J. Green (2004). *Health Promotion. Planning and Strategies.* London: SAGE.

Vike, H. (1996). Conquering the Unreal. Politics in a Norwegian Town. In: *Department and Museum of Anthropology.* Oslo: University of Oslo.

Vike, H. (1998). *Byråkratiske utopier. Antropologiske perspektiver på makt og kultur i offentlige organisasjoner.* Oslo: Institutt og museum for antropologi, Universitetet i Oslo.

Vike, H. (2004). *Velferd uten grenser 1. Den norske velferdsstaten ved veiskillet.* Oslo: Akribe.

Vike, H., Runar Bakken, Arne Brinchmann, Heidi Haukelien and Randi Kroken (eds.) (2002). *Maktens samvittighet. Om politikk, styring og dilemmaer i velferdsstaten*. Oslo: Gyldendal Akademisk.

WHO. (1948). *Constitution*. WHO, Geneva.

WHO. (1986). *Ottawa Charter of Health Promotion*. In: First International Conference on Health Promotion. Ottawa 17 – 21 November: WHO Regional Office in Europe, Copenhagen.

WHO. (1991). *Sundsvall Statement on Supportive Environment for Health*. In: The Third International Conference on Health Promotion. Sundsvall, Sweden: WHO Geneva.

WHO. (1997). *The Jakarta Declaration on Leading Health Promotion into the 21st Century*. In: The Fourth International Conference on Health Promotion. Jakarta, Indonesia: WHO, Geneva.

Young, A. (1995). *The Harmony of Illusions. Inventing Post-Traumatic Stress Disorder*. Princeton, NJ: Princeton University Press.

Anne-Lise Middelthon, Kåre Moen and Arne T. Høstmark

Chapter V.

# The silent life of good fatty tissue

Notions like 'bad fat' and 'good fat' are central in contemporary discourses on food and health. As semiotic resources, such concepts – and the distinction between them – make sense easily as long as we deal with non-human fat. In the realm of human fatty tissues, however, a different picture seems to emerge. With regard to fat as present in and on the body, on stomachs, on hips, on thighs etc., the good-bad distinction seems to make little sense in most health related discourses, be they lay or professional. Moreover, in these discourses, good fat such as olive oil and omega 3 may be good for your heart or brain, but never seems to do anything good for your fatty tissues. Some highly specialised bio-medical discourses in the fields of biochemistry and microbiology constitute an exception. Outside these discourses, however, human fatty tissue seems to be related to as inherently bad, unhealthy and dangerous to the person who embodies it, regardless of the quality of the fat incorporated by this very same person. Our concern here, then, is with phenomena related to the *qualities* of fat and how such qualities are dealt with or not dealt with in various discourses – scientific, lay, and public. This concern contrasts with the general emphasis on fat in terms of quantity or volume and/or, also, bodily location. On that note, it is worth stressing that our inquiry is conducted in the context of adipose tissue in normal and slightly overweight people. A discussion of phenomena which are *specifically* related to the *volume* of fatty tissues (such as problems associated with carrying a heavy mass of fat) falls outside the scope of the present discussion.

The inquiry of this paper was triggered by a brief exchange at a meeting at the Institute of General Practice and Community Medicine. [1] We start by giving an account of this event, and the questions it serendipitously gave rise to, and also of the way these questions were subsequently pursued. This paper is the result of a cross-disciplinary endeavour; Anne-Lise Middelthon is a social anthropologist, Arne T. Høstmark a medical doctor with special interest in physiology and biochemistry, and Kåre Moen a medical doctor with a background in general practice and international health. Such a multi-disciplinary approach allowed the subject under investigation to be explored from different angles. The structure of the paper reflects our process of inquiry in the sense that it offers separate accounts as well as jointly conducted discussions. Our working method is also reflected in our use of pronouns; starting off with I and me, evolving into we and us.

## The 'trigger' event

At a research meeting at our Institute the results from a population-based longitudinal study on body weight were presented (see Meyer and Tverdal, 2005). Among the issues that were brought up for debate was the question of how one should understand the coexistence of a significant increase in body mass index (BMI) among men over the past 30 years *and* (at the same time) a significant decrease in the risk of male cardiovascular disease. Running contrary to commonly held understandings about the relation between BMI and heart disease, the findings prompted questions such as whether this development might be due to the introduction of antihypertensive medication. This suggestion was discarded by the presenters. Then Arne, one of the authors of this chapter, remarked that if one also took into consideration that unsaturated fat had, to a large extent, replaced saturated fat as the preferred type of cooking fat in the observation period, an increased BMI combined with a decreased risk for cardiovascular disease might perhaps not be incompatible occurrences. This prompted Anne-Lise (also one of the authors) to ask: 'so, fat is not fat?'.[2] 'That is correct' Arne replied: 'the structure of the fat you eat will determine the structure of the body fat you get.'

The following first sections are Anne-Lise's account (related in first person) of how this brief exchange made it possible for her to catch sight of (some of) the implicit assumptions her understanding of such tissue had rested on. It is also an account of how serendipitous observations were turned into, and pursued as, research questions:

Before I move to the observations generated through the more systematic inquiry that followed the trigger event, let me dwell a little longer on the initial observations. Since cultural dimensions of food and feeding are my main field of research, I have of course dealt with fat, unsaturated and saturated types, perceptions of thinness and fatness, and so forth. Nevertheless, I had not before thought of fat as tissue whose structure *at cellular level* might differ from person to person and also change over time. Neither had I come across anybody who expressed such a take on fat until this meeting. Consequently I had never considered the possibility that fatty tissue might differ with regard to its effect on the health of the person who embodies it. The very idea that one lump of body fat might not be just another lump of body fat had simply not occurred to me. Unreflectedly, I had taken fat to be an undifferentiated body tissue whose structure would not differ from person to person. Hence, for me the knowledge I was confronted with at the meeting constituted a type of breach.[3] This breach or discontinuity made it possible for me to reconsider the notion of body fat that I unreflectedly had possessed and used until that moment,[4] i.e., it made it possible for me to reconsider the meaning of fat as a sign. Two characteristics of the sign, or notion, of fat which I hitherto had possessed came forth as particularly salient. First, this sign carried no (scientifically) informed knowledge about physical realities at cellular level. Second, this 'lack' was the kind of absence that is not recognised as such (an absence or lack). Concerning the latter, I had simply never self-consciously and critically reflected on the semiotic resources I had at my disposal for understanding 'fat' at the level of tissues and cells. In effect, I had taken myself to be sufficiently equipped to deal with this phenomenon. Of course, in order to identify an absence or lack there needs to be some idea of what is lacking, there needs to be some means of identifying the absence (Middelthon and Colapietro, 2005). And I had no such idea before Arne made his comment.

Significantly, despite the fact that the knowledge provided by Arne was radically new to me, his take on fatty tissue made immediate sense to me.

## Broadening the investigation

Already at the meeting mentioned above it was clear to me that I was not the only one who had held a notion of fat as a uniform and hence undifferentiated body tissue that in its structure did not vary much from human being to human being. While suspecting that harbouring such an understanding of human fatty tissue might not be limited to a few of us, I also realised that such a conclusion could not be taken for granted. The responses at the meeting had, however, indicated that to possess or not possess such knowledge about fatty tissue at the molecular level could not be reduced to a simple question of bio-medical versus more popular discourses.

The subsequent inquiry into the cultural and discursive dimensions of fatty tissue was pursued along two avenues. *First*, some of the questions triggered off by the event were immediately integrated into my ongoing research project, which focuses on the contemporary process of the medicalisation and instrumentalisation of food. By these terms I refer to a process through which food has come to find its main function as a means to achieve health-related goals. In this project, empirical data are generated through a combination of ethnographic methods: repeated exploratory interviews, group interviews,[5] analysis of mass media coverage of issues related to food and health, examination of popular and technical discourses on food and health, and participant observations in public meetings and at places where health and/or food are debated or in focus. In addition, since I am doing research 'at home', and the phenomena under scrutiny are encountered in countless everyday conversations, places, relations and contexts, the topics of inquiry inescapably become both external and internal to me as an investigator. For example, in the process of research, I (inevitably) began to pay special attention if the phenomenon of fat came up when I listened to people talk, read newspapers and professional journals, or looked at images and other forms of visualisations. Knowing that it was a topic that occupied me, others would bring it up in everyday conversations, just as I would.[6]

*Second* and as indicated above, as the inquiry undoubtedly would benefit from a multi-disciplinary approach, I invited both Arne (medical doctor with special interest in physiology and biochemistry) whose remarks had sparked off the inquiry, and Kåre (medical doctor with background in general practice and international health) to join me.

## First avenue of inquiry: the ongoing ethnographic research project

What kind of insights did integrating questions related to fatty tissue into the already ongoing ethnographic research project bring? The picture that soon emerged was that, to a large extent, people reacted in ways similar to mine. For example, in two focus groups among hospital staff and civil servants, respectively, no one had ever heard or thought of the possibility that fat, as a body tissue, was something that might differ from body to body, change over time, and potentially differ with its effect on the health of the person who embodied it. The same impression was found in discussions conducted with support groups consisting of women who had recently given birth to or adopted a child.

When offered an account of 'what Arne knew', namely, that the structure of a person's fatty tissues is not independent of the structure of the fat he or she has eaten, the response was surprisingly homogeneous. Significantly, despite expressing that they had never thought about fat in such a way before, all persons interacted with, with two exceptions only, also expressed (in one way or another) that this knowledge made sense to them. One of the two who disagreed, a student participating in a group discussion in a high school, downright rejected the idea that the structure of fat might differ from person to person dependent upon what they had been eating. Rather, she said, 'Fat is fat, no matter what!'

A historic parallel to how cholesterol had been perceived some years earlier was suggested in a project-related conversation with two high school teachers who teach subjects relevant to the project theme. After being introduced to the idea that fat is not necessarily a uniform tissue at cellular level, one of them replied:

> Yes, of course, that is how it must be. I have never before thought about it like that. That is indeed strange in itself. […] It was the same with cholesterol. Previously, cholesterol was also seen as one thing – a bad thing. The very idea that there might be both good and bad cholesterol was long resisted.

Through the conversation that followed it became clear that she was alluding to the possibility that conceptions of body fat as inherently bad might have to do with the status allocated to fat as a cultural phenomenon.

Before proceeding, it should be noted that even though the idea that fatty tissues may differ in structure was new to people, many mentioned that the localisation of fat on the body (hip versus abdomen) might be of significance with regard to health. Some also mentioned the production of estrogen in fat cells.

## Second avenue of inquiry: medical discourses

In the following section, Arne and Kåre, representing different medical disciplines, will in their technical discourses offer separate accounts of how fatty tissues are related to. From Arne's point of view, i.e. the specialised discourse of physiology and biochemistry, it is to state the obvious to say that what a person incorporates may determine the structural composition of his or her fatty tissues, and that such tissues (consequently) may differ from person to person and also change over time. Such knowledge forms a logical part of his take on how the human organism works and is self-evident to the degree that it is not even reflected on. By the tools of his specialised discourse Arne describes, in the following way, some aspects of the phenomenon under discussion:

Fatty acids are the main constituents of fats. They are energy substrates, precursors of cholesterol and hormones, serve as building material of cell membranes, and may influence membrane enzymes, hormone receptors, signal transduction, gene expression and growth (Jump, 2002; Jump and Clark, 1999). Fatty acids are released from adipose tissue in response to adrenergic stimulation, and are transported in the blood bound to a serum protein, albumin, from which the fatty acids are taken up in various tissues. Intake of fatty fish and fish oils may reduce the prevalence of cardiovascular events, some types of cancer, mental disorders, inflammatory diseases and possibly diabetes (Skerrett and Hennekens, 2003; Simopoulos, 2002; Augustsson et.al., 2003; Gil, 2002; Young and Conquer, 2005; Friedberg et.al., 1998). Such oils are rich in the long chain eicosapentaenoic (EPA, 20:5 ω3) and docosahexaenoic acids (DHA, 22:6 ω3). Physiologically, increased intake of fatty fish would provide more of these ω3-fatty acids to be used in various metabolic pathways, and for incorporation into the cell membranes, thereby influencing the many physiological processes mentioned above. Similarly, increased intake of other types of fat, e.g. butter fat, olive oil or rapeseed oil would alter the tissue composition and function accordingly. Importantly, fat in the body can be produced from excessive intake of carbohydrates, e.g. sugar, and this fat will be of the saturated type. Due to differences in diet, it would appear that the body fat composition may vary appreciably from society to society, and presumably also within a relatively homogeneous population. Thus, the fatty acid composition of the body (fat quality), including the adipose tissue, would govern the health risk. However, it is well established that severe overweight is associated with many diseases, such as diabetes and coronary heart diseases (e.g. Zalesin et al., 2008). (End of Arne's account).

If we move from Arne's specialised discourse of biochemistry to a more general bio-medical discourse, that of Kåre, a different picture emerges. Variations in molecular structure of fatty tissues do not seem to form an integral – or at least not a dominant or explicitly expressed – part of this discourse. Heterogeneity, in relation to body fat, is certainly a prominent theme but the main issue here seems to be volume and localisation; a question of *how much* and *where* on the body the tissue is located, *not* a question of *variations in the properties* of the fatty tissues. The following is Kåre's account:

That fatty tissue in any bodily position could potentially be 'good'? It did not immediately go down too well with me when the topic came up in a brief hallway chat. It would seem to mean that even 'belly fat' could potentially represent some degree of 'good', which seemed difficult to accept. My instincts told me that fat accumulating between and around abdominal organs was the ultimate example of fat that is always 'bad'.

As I often do when I want a quick indication that I am not totally out of touch, I ran a few quick web searches. I am an MD, but since I have not been in clinical medicine for some time I could easily have missed out on what 'everyone else' knows. What the search engines returned, however, was that colleagues were saying exactly the things I had expected. 'Belly fat' is 'the most dangerous kind of fat' (*USA Today*, 2008), 'has long been linked to an increased risk for insulin resistance and type 2 diabetes' (*HealthDay News*, 2008) and is 'much more damaging for the heart than a few extra pounds on your bottom, thighs and hips' (*Informationsdienst Wissenschaft*, 2008). Those at greatest risk are 'men whose waists are more than 40 inches in circumference and women whose waists are more than 35 inches in circumference' (ibid). Indeed, if 'your waist measurement is that high, you've fallen off the edge of the cliff' someone from Harvard was quoted as saying (*USA Today*, ibid). Still, the risk was not limited to those with big tummies, because 'although people who are overweight or obese are more likely to have large amounts of visceral fat, normal-weight people also can have too much' (ibid).

Except for the cliff simile, this was all too familiar to me. As expected, there seemed to be very little 'good' indeed to say about belly fat.

What neither I, nor the sources I had randomly consulted, factored into the picture, was the composition of visceral fat; its quality. It did not seem to strike us as particularly relevant whether a person's abdominal fat was the result of a diet rich in sugar or one rich in plant oils or fish fat. Although we would otherwise undoubtedly think of olive oil as much healthier than butter cookies, this did not seem to have a bearing on 'belly fat'.

For me – and I suspect for a number of other physicians and public health professionals – the potential harms of 'overweight' have been so high on the agenda for so long that 'fat' may have become close to synonymous with 'danger' for us. One might ask whether the construction of fat as a hazard has been so effective that we have rather limited room left for nuanced reflections about it. What fat signifies is risk for disability and death, full stop?

It is not, though, as if we never learnt that fat can (also) be a good thing.

As medical students we spent considerable amounts of time studying fat as part of our training in biochemistry and physiology. We learnt about the important, even essential, roles fat and fatty acids play in many bodily structures and functions. No human would be alive without bodily fat. No brain could work in its absence. Several vitamins could not be absorbed if there was none around.

Although fat is clearly part of the amazing body, I suspect few of us have spent much time after medical school reflecting on the marvels of it. The following snippet from the WHO website, on the other hand, feels rather fully internalised in me:

> Obesity has reached epidemic proportions globally, with more than 1 billion adults overweight – at least 300 million of them clinically obese – and is a major contributor to the global burden of chronic disease and disability. [...] Obesity is a complex condition, with serious social and psychological dimensions, affecting virtually all ages and socioeconomic groups. (WHO, 2008)

One is in no doubt that it is a grave public health enemy that is described in this text, with its remarkable figures and fairly dramatic wording. It could arguably be interpreted as the manifesto on which the war on fat is founded. In that war, it is primarily quantities and locations that matter. What we are combating are amounts and volumes.

The focus on quantities is also reflected in the tools that have been commonly used to advise people about food, fat and exercise. The Body Mass Index (BMI) evaluates a person's weight in relation to his or her height. If the weight divided by the height squared is above 25.0, the person is classified as 'overweight'. If it is above 30.0, s/he is considered 'obese'. Together with a measurement of the person's waist circumference, these BMI-related classifications of people are, in turn, linked to explicit predictions about individual disease risk. And the relationship between BMI, waist circumference and disease risk has normally been presented as (remarkably) simple, clear and strong, as in this familiar table (National Heart, Lung and Blood Institute, 2008).

## Classification of Overweight and Obesity by BMI, Waist Circumference and Associated Disease Risks

*Disease Risk\* Relative to Normal Weight and Waist Circumference+*

| | BMI (kg/m²) | Obesity Class | Men 102 cm (40 in) or less Women 88 cm (35 in) or less | Men > 102 cm (40 in) Women > 88 cm (35 in) |
|---|---|---|---|---|
| Underweight | < 18.5 | | – | – |
| Normal | 18.5 – 24.9 | | – | – |
| Overweight | 25.0 – 29.9 | | Increased | High |
| Obesity | 30.0 – 34.9 | I | High | Very High |
| | 35.0 – 39.9 | II | Very High | Very High |
| Extreme Obesity | 40.0 + | III | Extremely High | Extremely High |

\* Disease risk for type 2 diabetes, hypertension, and CVD.

+ Increased waist circumference can also be a marker for increased risk even in persons of normal weight.

Effectively, height, weight and waist circumference appears to be all you need to determine at what level of risk a person is for three significant diseases: diabetes, hypertension and cardiovascular disease (CVD). Not even in a footnote is the picture complicated with reflections about the quality of the fat a person ingests or harbours.[7]

I grew up as a professional with this table. It was my ABC. Still surprised that I hesitated that day in the hallway?

## Discussion

From different angles and perspectives, the three of us have discussed the phenomenon that, except from some highly specialised bio-medical discourses such as biochemistry and microbiology, human fatty tissues seem to be related to as tissues that are intrinsically bad. A distinction between bad and good fat does not seem to apply to human fat cells and fatty tissues in (most) lay and public health discourses on fat and health. A related phenomenon is found in the way that claims about the effects of good fat on the human body are expressed (it should again be noted that this is radically different from the way such effects are articulated in micro-biological and bio-chemical discourses). In public health and lay discourses, statements about the effect of good fat such as olive oil and fish oils tend to be articulated in ways like these: 'olive oil is good for your body' or 'olive oil is good for *the* body', as well as 'olive oil is good for your heart, 'omega-3 is good for your brain' or 'cod liver oil will improve the intelligence of your child'. Such statements are easily encountered in everyday conversations, mass media, public health messages and clinical consultations and will normally evoke little, if any, controversy. At least two features of this way of relating to the health-related effects of fat come forth as being of interest to the discussion. First, the beneficial effects of good fat seem either to be linked to the body as a generalised entity (it is good for 'your body' or 'the body'), or directly to one specific organ or function (it is good for your 'brain' or 'heart'). Second, if the latter claims (those that link the effect of good fat to one specific function or organ) are scrutinised as a package and we thereby gain an opportunity to identify what is not part of this parcel, at least one lack or absence becomes apparent: *There is a lack of any claim about (any potential) beneficial effect of good fat on fatty tissues or fat cells.* The good fat we eat may be good for a number of organs and functions but never seems to be of any good for the fatty tissues we have, or get.[8] This absence of the potential good effects of fat on fat becomes even more intriguing if one considers that such claims are not wanting when it comes to non-human beings (such as fish). Recent research reporting, that the fat of farmed salmons becomes better and healthier when good oil/fat is added to the fodder of such fish, has been received as almost self explanatory (Seierstad, 2008).

While a distinction between bad and good seems to make no sense at the level of human fatty tissue, such a distinction makes perfectly good sense when it comes to the classification of food and foodstuffs for human beings. Here, the concepts of 'bad fat' (such as butter) and 'good fat' (such as olive oil) form an integral part of common classification schemes (e.g. Middelthon, 2006). If the general acceptance of an existence of good as well as bad fat-foodstuff for human consumption and incorporation is considered together with the omnipresence of sayings like 'you are what you eat' (a saying which comes forth almost as a truism to most of us),[9] questions like the following may easily arise: How can it be that neither our capacity to meaningfully differentiate between good and bad fat (in the food we do or do not eat), nor our apparent agreement with the statement that 'we are what we eat', are extended to fat at cellular level? Why is it that this logic seemingly does not apply to human body fat? Why does the good fat we incorporate never materialise as (visible) good fat on the body?

If one is to make an attempt to answer such questions, it will of course not suffice to limit the field of inquiry to the realm of health and illness. On the contrary, 'fat' will need to be considered in the larger cultural context of its operation. In that context, human body fat is not only regarded as ugly and unattractive but also as tissues that possess a capacity to reveal something about the character of the person who embodies it. As discussed by many; too much fat is seen as a sign of lack of self-restraint and self-control, and hence a weakness of will and dubious moral (For example Gard and Wright 2005 and Throsby 2007).[10] This association between fat and moral laxity, and lack of will power, forms part of the cultural framework many of us, habitually and unreflectedly, draw upon when we make inferences about fat and fatty tissues. Within this framework fat is also increasingly being perceived as a sign of being a bit dumb, poor and belonging to the lower strata of society. Furthermore, fat is not only seen as an evil for the person who embodies it but also for society at large and its economy. In sum, fat is simply not something one wants to be associated with; human fatty tissues are not (culturally) associable with anything good – at least not with regard to health, will and morality.

Human fatty tissues are, in many ways, related to as tissues that don't really belong to the body. The splitting off of fatty tissue from the general logic governing incorporation of fat (as discussed above) may be seen as one expression of such an (implicit) cultural notion of fat. Through this exclusion, body fat oddly acquires an almost extra-bodily status. Making body fat into something *other* than the rest of the body, seems to form part of how the general cultural take on fat is construed. Within this framework, fat seems indeed to be implicitly at work as the body's other. By such an othering of body fat, a distance is also made to its attributed meanings; the lack of will and the bad moral.

But this should not be taken to mean that such a take on fat is not amendable. On the contrary – and as described above – when exposed to the logic of the discourse within which Arne works (bio-chemistry and physiology), the people interacted with typically reacted by saying that they had never heard or thought about fat in this way before. Their reaction, however, did not stop there. Most added almost immediately (in various phrasings, of course) that this new knowledge nevertheless made perfectly good sense to them (the structure of the fat you eat will have consequences for the structure of the fat you get, where ever on your body it might be found). Their reaction testifies not only to the need to critically reflect on the signs and frameworks at our disposal but also to the need to do so in dialogue with frameworks other than those we normally work, and think, within, and in relation to. To do so may be especially pertinent when dealing with phenomena associated with cultural rejection and even disgust.

Lastly, Mark Graham coined the term 'lipoliteracy'[11] to designate our capacity to read fat: "In fat-obsessed cultures we are all 'lipoliterates' who 'read' fat for what we believe it tells us about a person. This includes not only their moral character but also their health" (2005: 178-79). As we have tried to show, the scope of our lipoliteracy, our ability to read fat, seems fairly circumscribed and restricted. This paper is a modest attempt to make a contribution to efforts that aims at making us slightly more literate in the field of fat, and fatty tissues.

## Notes

1 The authors are all based at the Institute of General Practice and Community Medicine at the Faculty of Medicine, University of Oslo: Arne T. Høstmark is a Professor at the Institute's Section for Preventive Medicine, whereas Kåre Moen is a Research Fellow and Anne-Lise Middelthon an Associate Professor at its Section for Medical Anthropology and Medical History.

2 'Så [kropps] fett er ikke [kropps] fett.'

3 A self-conscious realisation of this kind is by necessity also an observation of what one knows now and what one did not know before.

4 With Foucault (for example, 1999 [1971]; this incidence changed the 'conditions of possibility' for my understanding and experience of fatty tissues and hence fat as a more generalised phenomenon. (Since, this paper is informed by semiotics in the Peircean tradition, this is an example of a generation of an interpretant that is radically different from the one preceding it in the semiotic process – or semiosis).

5 Repeated exploratory interviews have been conducted with persons who had previously participated in a comprehensive population-based study in Oslo. Group-interviews are being conducted with persons in south-east Norway who are in some way already connected and share an everyday reality that involves food (for example, groups of women who have recently given birth, people who eat lunch together at work, elderly people who eat at centres for elderly, people who meet as neighbours, schoolmates).

6 While doing anthropology at home is recognised as a circumstance that may supply depth and texture to the research material generated through more formal means, it is also recognised as a continuous challenge demanding a carefully considered, and ceaseless, alternation between productive closeness and the necessary distance to the field.

7 It is emphasised, however, that for some athletes the BMI may not at all reflect the amount of fat in the body, and this is well known among researchers.

8 As noted above, one exception may be found in the relatively recent recognition of good fat as being good for the cholesterol in our blood.

9 Of course, since Roland Barthes'(1979[1961]) classical consideration of the capacity of food to function as signs which mark and produce social and cultural distinctions, and hence identities and difference, a rich volume of general and local studies and analyses has been generated. But the particular association between food and identity is not the theme here.

10 To see fat as linked to the character of a person is not only a contemporary phenomenon. (See for example Guerrini, 2000; Lupton, 1996).

11 Mark Graham (2005:178) makes his analysis of cultural readings of fat in the contexts of lipodystrophy as a side effect of HAART (Highly Active Anti-Retroviral Therapy).

## Bibliography

Augustsson, K., Michaud D.S., Rimm, E.B., Leitzmann, M.F., Stampfer, M.J., Willett, W.C. and Giovannucci, E. (2003). A prospective study of intake of fish and marine fatty acids and prostate cancer. *Cancer Epidemiology, Biomarkers & Prevention*, 12, 64-67.

Barthes, R. (1979) [1961]. *Annales*, vol. 5 (Trans. Forster and Ranum). Baltimore and London: The Johns Hopkins University Press.

Foucault, M. (1999) [1971]. *Diskursens orden* (L'ordre de Discours, translated into English as The Discourse of Language). Oslo: Spartacus Forlag.

Friedberg, C.E., Janssen, M.J., Heine, R.J. and Grobbee, D.E. (1998). Fish oil and glycemic control in diabetes. A meta-analysis. *Diabetes Care*, 21, 494-500.

Gil, A. (2002). Polyunsaturated fatty acids and inflammatory diseases. *Biomedicine and Pharmacotherapy*, 56, 388-396.

Guerrini, A. (2000). *Obesity & Depression in the Enlightment. The Life and Times of George Cheyne*. University of Oklahoma Press.

Graham, M. (2005). Chaos. In: Meneley A. and Kulich D. (eds.). *Fat: the anthropology of an obsession*. New York, J.P. Tarcher/Penguin.

*HealthDay News*: Blood Test Warns of Dangerous 'Deep Belly' Fat. http://yourtotal-health.ivillage.com/blood-test-warns-dangerous-deep-belly-fat.html. Accessed 22.09.2008.

*Informationsdienst Wissenschaft*: Exercise is the best medicine for dangerous abdominal obesity. http://idw-online.de/pages/de/news216609. Accessed 22.09.2008.

Jump, D.B. and Clarke, S.D. (1999). Regulation of gene expression by dietary fat. *Annual Review of Nutrition*, 19, 63-90.

Jump, D.B. (2002). The biochemistry of n-3 polyunsaturated fatty acids. *The Journal of Biological Chemistry*, 277, 8755-8758.

Lupton, D. (1996). *Food, the Body and the Self*. London: Sage Publications.

Meyer, H.E. and Tverdal, A. (2005). Development of body weight in the Norwegian population. In: *Prostaglandins, Leukotrienes and Essential Fatty Acids*, 73, 3-7.

Middelthon, A-L and Colapietro, V. (2005). Absent Signs, Elusive Experience: on young gay men and absence of adequate signs and cultural images. In: Lee, Lanice W. (ed.). *Psychology of Gender Identity*. New York: Nova Science Publisher.

Middelthon, A-L. (2006). Farmakologisering av mat. *Nytt Norsk Tidsskrift*, 3, 261-68.

National Heart Lung and Blood Institute: Classification of Overweight and Obesity by BMI, Waist Circumference and Associated Disease Risks. http://www.nhlbi.nih.gov/health/public/heart/obesity/lose_wt/bmi_dis.htm. Accessed 22.09.2008.

Seierstad, S.L. (2008). *The effect on fish and human health of replacing marine oils by vegetable oils in feeds of Atlantic salmon*. Norwegian School of Veterinary Science.

Simopoulos, A.P. (2002). Omega-3 fatty acids in inflammation and autoimmune diseases. *Journal of the American College of Nutrition*, 21, 495-505.

Skerrett, P.J. and Hennekens, C.H. (2003). Consumption of fish and fish oils and decreased risk of stroke. *Preventive Cardiology*, 6, 38-41.

Throsby, K. (2007). "How could you let yourself get like that?": Stories of the origins of obesity in accounts of weight loss surgery. *Social Science & Medicine* 65 (8): 1561-1571.

*USA Today*: Belly full of danger. http://www.usatoday.com/news/health/2003-02-25-bellyfat-usat_x.htm. Accessed 22.09.2008.

WHO: Global Strategy on Diet, Physical Activity and Health. http://www.who.int/dietphysicalactivity/publications/facts/obesity/en/. Accessed 22.09.2008.

Young G. and Conquer, J. (2005). Omega-3 fatty acids and neuropsychiatric disorders. *Reproduction, Nutrition, Development* 2005, 45, 1-28.

Zalesin K.C., Franklin B.A., Miller W.M., Peterson E.D. and McCullough P.A. (2008). Impact of obesity on Cardiovascular disease. *Endocrinology and Metabolism Clinics of North America*, 37, 663-84.

Sjaak van der Geest[1]

Chapter VI.

# Patients as co-researchers? Views and experiences in Dutch medical anthropology

## Introduction

In this paper I want to raise questions about developments in medical anthropology in my own country The Netherlands. Is Dutch medical anthropology undergoing changes as a result of a shift in power between the healthcare system, patients / clients and the world of research, in particular medical anthropology? Is there a shift from anthropology *of* to anthropology *in* medicine, to use the old distinction? In her contribution to this volume, Sylvie Fainzang warns us that we should not let ourselves be co-opted by biomedicine, as we have our own anthropological perspective. Another development may be equally – or more – relevant here: the rising power of patient organisations in the negotiations of healthcare policy and research. Patients / clients / care consumers now present themselves as candidates for doing or sharing research that deals with *their* wellbeing. How does this trend affect 'medical anthropology at home'?

I will first briefly sketch the rise of patient consciousness and then argue that this development dovetails with the central principles of anthropological research. The main body of my presentation will be an overview and discussion of trends in this field within The Netherlands, and how these events affect medical anthropology. In my conclusion I will address why the rise of patient movements did not – or hardly – affect medical anthropological research in Dutch academia.

## Rise of patient consciousness

The increased awareness among patients of their rights and their specific experiences *as* patients is well known and has been extensively documented. In 2003 the *British Medical Journal* (*BMJ*) introduced a theme issue titled 'The patient', where a number of distinguished scholars, policy-makers and practitioners pleaded for more 'patient-centred' medicine. The then editor Richard Smith wrote in his editorial:

> ... being patient centred involves much more than being dedicated and caring. It's a different way of thinking and behaving, where doctors and patients work together as true partners. (Smith, 2003:1274)

The theme issue explored the meanings and implications of 'true partnership' and looked ahead to a time that the journal – a typical doctors' journal – might be a common enterprise of doctors and patients (nurses are not mentioned). In 1997 *BMJ* invited a patient to join its editorial board. A few years later it started a website about 'best treatments' for doctors as well as for patients. Around 2003 *BMJ* appointed a patient editor, Mary Baker. The objective of this theme issue, Smith wrote, was "to help doctors prepare for a world where true partnership with patients is the norm" (Smith, 2003: 1274).

The rise of patient power is of course closely related to the consumer movement. An example of how a consumer organisation develops into a patient, or – more 'correctly' – a health consumer movement is the British organisation Involve, which promotes the involvement of consumers in decision-making regarding services and policy.[2]

The term 'patient' is itself a symbol of the passive and powerless position of people who face health or disability problems. Blume and Catshoek (2003: 183-184) criticise the term as misleading (and offensive, I would add). Why should someone be called a 'patient', if he / she is deaf or using a wheelchair but hardly ever sees a doctor? Still, even *if* he frequents the doctor, why the term 'patient'? The patient stereotype is well described by Cayton:

> Anxious, weak, perhaps in pain and deprived of clothes, usually cowed into submission by lengthy waiting, and almost always ignorant of what is wrong with us and what will happen to us. We are hardly in a position to be active consumers. You cannot be an active consumer without the power of information. (Blume and Catshoek, 2003: 183)

In the Dutch context, however, terms like 'consumer' or 'client' are less common. There is some resistance to their euphemistic cover-up and most organisations continue to call themselves 'patient organisations'.[3] The term 'patient' almost assumes the status of a self-applied nickname, a *geuzen-*

*naam*, as it is called in Dutch. For the rest, the patient movement in The Netherlands does not seem to be very different from what occurs in the United Kingdom. The organisations mainly focus on advocacy, furthering the interests of their members and building a more 'normal' image and social identity of people with a sickness or disability (cf., Duyvendak and Nederland, 2007).

I will focus here on one of the objectives of patient organisations: to get actively involved in research that deals with *them*. That ambition follows logically from the wish to have their share in decision-making on policy and services and from their growing self-consciousness: they are convinced that they have knowledge that is crucial for carrying out scientific research that 'normal' researchers lack. In Dutch we speak of *ervaringskennis* (experiential knowledge) and *ervaringsdeskundigheid* (experiential expertise). It is here that medical anthropology enters.

## Medical anthropology

One does not need to convince an anthropologist that the views and experiences of a sick or disabled person matter when studying sickness or disability. That insight lies at the heart of anthropological research. Our insistence on the emic point of view is in fact an invitation to sick and disabled persons to speak about their experiences. Participation, our hallmark, is an attempt to come as closely as possible to the lived experience of those we study. Intersubjectivity is a prerequisite for doing anthropological research (cf., Tankink and Vysma, 2006). Without sharing subjectivity, ethnography remains stale and unconvincing. The importance we attach to the views and experiences of those we study shows in our writing: we favour long quotations and narratives from our informants and repeatedly state that we want to give them a voice.

That concern to capture *their* point of view continues during the writing-up. Many of us show what we have written to our informants and ask for comments and corrections (cf., Stoller, 1985). At the same time, we explicitly demonstrate our awareness that we will never fully capture their views. By using the first person singular we acknowledge that in the end it is still *I* who writes, interprets and draws conclusions. We admit the limitations of our intersubjectivity (cf., Estroff, 1995).

The idea of active involvement of patients (or other interested parties) in the planning, conducting and writing up of research goes far beyond what Fisher (1986) calls 'collaborating informants' or what Marcus (1999) terms 'circumstantial activism'. It also differs fundamentally from yet another methodological concept 'complicity' (Homes, 1993; Marcus, 1997, 1998).

'Complicity' refers to the engagement of a researcher in a relationship with informants who are involved in dubious or illicit business. A classic, but rather innocent example is Geertz's entanglement in an illegal cockfight in Bali (Geertz 1973b). It is an affinity that comes into existence in the field and does indeed lead to more intersubjectivity and, therefore, to better ethnography. It does not, however, include the control over each phase of the research, as is envisaged in the patient-induced research. A similar comment can be made regarding the concept of 'collaborating informants', which demonstrates the transactional nature of ethnographic knowledge. Using a case by Crapanzano (1980), Fisher shows that the involvement of an informant as collaborator helps him to see his own knowledge as:

> ... more subtly constructed through the action of others. Our knowledge is shown to be less objective, more negotiated by human interests ... (1986: 208)

'Circumstantial activism', coined by Marcus (1999), is also primarily a methodological technique. Its purpose is to improve the epistemological quality of a research. It is a 'modest intervention' that helps to conceptualise the problems that are being addressed in the research project (cf., Hine, 2007: 656).

It is no wonder that medical anthropological studies that have been written by patients are particularly cherished. We believe that these authors are in a privileged position to understand suffering and we acknowledge their authority.

Well-known examples of researchers who were affected by a serious sickness and used their experience to write more empathically (and more intelligently) about illness are Arthur Frank (1995), Irving Zola (1982) and Robert Murphy (1988).[4] Murphy writes about his illness over a period of eighteen years, from the moment the first symptoms of a spinal cord tumour presented themselves to his being restricted to a wheelchair and becoming dependent on others. This ethnography about one person shows what illness does to social identity. His struggle for autonomy slowly grows into acceptance and discovery of deeper meanings. His reflection starts with an observation when he still was an outsider to the world of disease and disability. He sees a severely disabled person in a wheelchair and wonders why such a person would want to live. He is unable to grasp that person's desire for life. When, many years later, he is disabled himself, he remembers that moment and is finally able to explain to himself and his readers how much life still holds for him.

Frank (1995, 2001) has written extensively about his own illness experiences, using them as 'data' that enhance his authority as an author of sickness and suffering. Suffering is what cannot be spoken about (Frank, 2001). He takes the position of a patient who is approached by a researcher. That meeting can lead to feelings of disrespect and insult if the sick person feels he/she is broken down into ethnographically and theoretically interesting fragments. Estroff reports a similar incident (1995). She begins her article with an angry informant who has read her story in the anthropologist's book and feels 'exploited'. Similarly, Kleinman and Kleinman (1991) criticised anthropologists for transforming illness experiences into academic anthropological concepts.

A less known example of a patient who became (or rather remained) a researcher is Gerhard Nijhof, a medical sociologist, who was diagnosed with cancer and underwent surgery. He spent an anxious period in the hospital and had to learn how to live with his disease. Being critically ill was not a matter of being 'patient' but of hard work. The cancer changed his life *and* his sociology. *Ziekenwerk* [Sick work], the short book he wrote about his experiences, is an attempt, from an insider's perspective, to forge a new kind of medical sociology (Nijhof, 2001). For most medical sociologists, he writes, serious illness is not a personal experience. They conduct surveys or hold interviews and return to their universities or homes to analyse and write their findings. The concepts they use reveal their provenance: the minds of healthy sociologists. Nijhof became acutely aware of this when he fell sick, encountering completely different concepts.

One such concept was the *unspoken* word. For years he had been studying words, spoken and written ones. Analyses of texts had been his main occupation, but he came to realise that people may remain silent about certain experiences. 'Yet, we continue to pay attention to their speaking only … the things about which they don't speak escape us.' That is the reason why 'interrogating sociologists miss so much of what sickness means to sick people.' A sickness such as cancer is mainly surrounded by silence. The contribution by Els van Dongen to this volume is yet another illustration of the authority and cogency that one has when quoting from one's own experience of pain and uncertainty.

Writing from one's own experience enhances the validity and reliability. I speak of 'validity' if my conversation partner (or 'informant') understands my question and if his response is indeed an answer to what I meant to ask.

Knowing with a reasonable amount of certainty that we understand each other and are able to exchange our views on an issue that we both – again, with a reasonable amount of certainty – see in the same way is, after all, a result of intersubjectivity. Such intersubjectivity is built upon and develops during a sequence of meetings and conversations. During a brief and only encounter between an *enquêteur* and a respondent, intersubjectivity is unlikely to occur or – at most – remains an unknown factor (cf., Bleek, 1987).

Similar remarks can be made with regard to reliability, which I understand in its everyday meaning. Are the informant's answers frank and trustworthy? Or does he try to hide information? 'Lying informants' are common; why should someone tell the truth about something that is not the other person's business? And why should he offend the researcher by refusing to give an answer? Giving an 'other' answer may be a more polite and convenient solution in such a situation (cf., Van Dongen and Fainzang, 2005). 'Lying' is meaningful, as Salamone (1977) once remarked. When people lie, it usually means that something important is at stake. Lucky is the researcher who stumbles upon a lying informant. The problem, however, is that one first needs to know when lying or concealment takes place. Again, it is only by intersubjectivity and circumstantial evidence (Geertz, 1973a: 23) that we are able to sense this.

Obviously, where researcher and research subject have a common interest, as is advocated by patient organisations, lying or concealment will be quite useless and misunderstanding (in-validity) less likely.

Finally, taking research one-step further toward policy-making and practical service, only valid and reliable information will produce meaningful and useful suggestions for health – and healthy – care problems. Meaningfulness is crucial because policy needs to take the perceptions and experiences of patients as the starting point, and usefulness is necessary because policy must address the problems of patients (and not those of other stakeholders).

In conclusion, the 'philosophy' of (medical) anthropology seems particularly apt to embrace the active involvement of patients in all phases of a research: in its preparation, execution, analysis and application. Let us now look at how the idea of patients as co-researchers was launched in The Netherlands and how medical anthropologists reacted to this idea.

## Discussions and experiments in The Netherlands

In 2001 the Dutch organisation PatiëntenPraktijk commissioned Stuart Blume and Geerke Catshoek to write a report about the possibility of including patient organisations in scientific research. Their report suggested three strategies to achieve this objective:

- Bring about structures for dialogue between scientists and patient organisations;
- Strengthen the legitimacy of patient participation in research;
- Promote and develop new styles of research (Blume and Catshoek, 2001).

All three recommendations were already common practice in medical anthropology, so the report provided an excellent opportunity to test the principles of medical anthropology and to place the anthropological approach in the spotlight of Dutch healthcare research.

We invited Blume and Catshoek to write a 'teaser' for the annual symposium of the journal *Medische Antropologie* (Blume and Catshoek, 2003). The symposium on 'The role of patients in research' was held in December 2003. Six months later, seven papers that had been presented at the symposium, plus one that had been added, were published in a special issue of the journal under the title 'The patient as co-researcher.' Interestingly, only two of these contributions had actually been authored – or co-authored – by a 'patient.' None of them reported on the outcome of a research that had been carried out jointly by professional and patient researchers.

Let us look more closely at some of these publications. The first article (Klop et al., 2004) presented the policy of the national fund for healthcare research, ZonMw, to enhance the interaction between researchers and patients. The article was written by three (non-patient) representatives of the funding programme.

The second article by a 'patient' volunteer for the Dutch League of Arthritis Patients Associations (De Wit, 2004) highlighted the obstacles he had encountered when he tried to promote the patient perspective among researchers. Like the first one, this contribution developed ideas on how patients could play a role in research; it did not show any results of such research.

An article by Abma et al. (2004) did report on a research that was carried out in close cooperation between professional researchers and members of a paraplegia association. One of the authors was a paraplegia patient. The article discussed methodological and strategic aspects, rather than the outcome of the research.

The last example is an article that described an experiment with older people (over 85) who were asked to comment on, and possibly correct, the outcome of a research on 'successful ageing' in a Dutch provincial town (Von Faber 2004). The results of the research, which was a combined qualitative and quantitative study, had been published in a booklet in comprehensible language and large print, which had been distributed among all (almost 600) participants of the research. Out of 320 participants that were invited to take part in the discussion, only 21 responded. I was myself involved in the group discussions and vividly remember the disappointing results of the meetings. We had clearly over-estimated the ability of these older people to critically assess the findings and conclusions of the research. They mainly came to thank us or to ask a question. One man produced a sheet of paper and started to give a formal speech in praise of the research team. Six of the participants had never read the booklet or did not even remember they had received a copy. Others vaguely remembered they had read it but did not know the contents anymore. Our expectations of critical comments proved indeed unrealistic and I began to doubt about the feasibility of some forms of patient-led research. Sometimes, it seems, it is the professional rather than the patient who insists on patient participation.

A few months after the publication of the special issue on 'The patient as co-researcher', ZonMw, the Dutch national fund, organised an 'after-noon study' for patient organisations. About seventy people attended. Five speakers and a lively plenary discussion addressed conditions, possibilities and examples of research projects that involved patients as co-researchers. The meeting produced a list of 21 recommendations to enhance patient-research, most of which were of a practical nature such as training patient-researchers, digital support, communication, and payment.

This type of afternoon study has since been held every year. The meetings have stimulated and inspired patient organisations and individual patient-researchers. A team of patient-researchers and non-patient profes-sionals also wrote a handbook for patient participation in scientific research (Smit et al., 2006). It provides a wealth of practical suggestions on how and where the contribution of a patient-researcher could be most valuable: evaluation of research proposal, patient information, style of interview-ing, mediating between researcher and patient population, monitoring of research, analysing data, and distributing results (Smit et al., 2006: 20).

The handbook also contains vignettes with concrete examples of the various possibilities and pitfalls of patient research. Another handbook on patient participation appeared one year later (Abma and Broerse, 2007). The authors are a management specialist and a medical biologist. Two years earlier Caron-Flinterman, a specialist in Science and Technology Studies, defended her dissertation on patient participation in decision-making on biomedical research. Her starting point was that 'stakeholders participation' seemed an increasingly common phenomenon in healthcare research but not in basic biomedical research. The main question of her study, therefore, was to what extent patient participation would be possible in decision-making concerning biomedical research.

More activities and publications could be mentioned here, but I will leave it at this (for a now, somewhat dated, Dutch overview, see Smit 2005). The point I want to make is that after we drew attention to the advantage of having patient-researchers, this idea has gradually drifted away from medical anthropology and moved toward medical and behavioural scientists. Medical anthropologists have hardly played a role in the developments that have taken place since. Why?

## Medical anthropological silence

Before I try to account for the apparent loss of interest among medical anthropologists to engage in joint research with patient-colleagues, let me recount one attempt to bring these two parties together. During the discussions on the first afternoon study, I told the representatives of the various patient organisations that some of our medical anthropology and sociology students were searching for topics for their master research. I suggested that I could mediate between them and the students to find research topics that both parties would find relevant and that could be researched in mutual cooperation. They reacted positively. I wrote to 40 organisations explaining my willingness to broker a suitable research topic for the students and asked them to formulate one or more questions they deemed relevant and to name a person in their organisation who was willing to participate in the research. Fifteen organisations responded. Most of them listed a question they wanted to study or indicated that they would decide on a question in consultation with the student. I distributed the information from the organisations among the students and waited for their reactions.

The reactions were minimal. Out of forty students who were planning to participate in this joint research, only one got involved with a patients' organisation, an association of people suffering from chronic pain. One of the activities of the association was to organise training sessions to help people coping with continuous pain. They wanted to know if their sessions were successful; how they had affected the lives of the participants; if they had improved the quality of their lives; and if the participants now used less medication for their pain.

These questions were largely typical for most questions that patient organisations wanted to address: practical issues that had direct relevance for their work. I suspect that the students' lukewarm reaction can be partly explained by the practical nature of the questions that the organisations suggested. They appeared uninteresting and too thin for students who wanted to write an anthropological thesis. How could they devote an academic discussion to such simple questions? They rather seemed questions for an evaluation questionnaire.

The student who did connect with a patient organisation eventually wrote a thesis on the expectations people with chronic pain have toward the organisation (Schrama, 2006).

## Conclusion: Uneasy bedfellows

Let me now try to offer a few possible reasons why patient organisations and medical anthropologists are less easy bedfellows than one might expect. And particularly: why so little research takes place between anthropologists and patient-researchers.

One reason may be that patients and medical anthropologists have different interests after all. Patients and their organisations are mainly focused on very practical matters – mostly medical and financial ones – that alleviate their problems such as pain and restrictions on treatment. Improvement of medical facilities and medication are probably the most outspoken ones. Research that serves their interests and which they want to promote and influence will therefore be largely in the field of biomedicine. Caron-Flinterman (2005: 105-116) who listed the most urgent problems among patients with Asthma and Chronic Obstructive Pulmonary Disease (COPD) confirms this. Their two, by far most urgent, problems were 'side-effects of medication' and 'hypersensitivity for all kinds of substances.' Social aspects of their problems, such as 'interference with social life', 'inadequate collaboration of healthcare professionals' and 'non-understanding by social environment' proved much less urgent. Their priorities for research largely reflected the above list. The author concludes that the patients 'prioritised biomedical research – research on the aetiology of the diseases and on new and better medication – above research on healthcare, social, or political issues' (p. 112).

Clearly, medial anthropological research is less 'interesting' for patients: it does not address their main concerns. Moreover, the social problems that patients did prioritise, hardly interest anthropological researchers. They are often considered too simple and too practical to carry out research that will be appreciated in anthropological circles. Anthropologists may claim that they are led by 'what really matters' to the patient (cf. Kleinman 2006) but in actual fact what matters to *them* is more likely to direct them in their research. What matters to them is rich ethnography (good stories) and theoretical innovation. Kleinman and Kleinman remark that:

> What is lost in biomedical renditions – the complexity, uncertainty and or-
> dinariness of some man or woman's unified world of experience – is also
> missing when illness is reinterpreted as social role, social strategy, or social
> symbol ... anything but human experience ... Ethnography does participate
> in this professional transformation of an experience-rich and -near human
> subject into a dehumanised object, a caricature of experience. (1991: 276)

Instead of capturing their point of view and their experience, anthropologists may thus turn patients into objects of metaphorisation and academic debate and miss the point they set out to make. As a result – and ironically – medical doctors and biomedical researchers may be closer to patients and their interests than anthropologists who have made it their business to be close to them. Or am I now too optimistic about the medical profession?

A second reason, related to the previous one, may be that the idea of co-researching derives more from the anthropologist's search for epistemological legitimacy and advanced methodology than from the patient's strife for better living conditions. In other words, anthropologists may be interested in patients who play an active role during fieldwork and in the writing-up period because this produces better ethnography and anthropology. Patients may thus be used for the benefit of anthropological ambitions. It is not surprising then that the co-operation between patient- and anthropological researchers does not really materialise.

Thirdly, some anthropologists will look upon patient-led research with suspicion. Patient-led research is supposed to lead to applied research, which has never been fully accepted in mainstream anthropology. The old adage of non-intervention still holds strong, be it in a more subtle form than before. Small interventions in the everyday life of fieldwork are accepted and have become a normal part of the methodological canon of participatory observation. However, research that has been explicitly designed to be applied and make the world better is as suspect as it was fifty years ago among the majority of anthropologists.

Even 'icons' of critical medical anthropology (such as – in alphabetic order – Baer, Estroff, Farmer, Fassin, Inhorn, Kaufman, Kleinman, Lock, Mattingly, Nichter and Scheper-Hughes), who explicitly state that their research is to change the wrongs and inequality in health and healthcare, did not invite patients as equal co-researchers. Patients and their fellow-sufferers are quoted extensively in the publications but further does their contribution not go.

In conclusion, in spite of a remarkable affinity between the anthropological 'philosophy' of patient-centred and experience-near research on the one side and patients' interest in direct involvement in research on the other, the two parties hardly succeed in actually doing joint research. Anthropologists will have to give up some of their most cherished theoretical and methodological prerequisites to turn their on-paper interests in patient-led research into actual practice. Moreover, they should take into account that there may be more 'theory' hiding in the 'simple' questions that patient organisations raise than they – somewhat prematurely – assume. I am afraid, however, that only a small and somewhat marginal minority in medical anthropology is likely to take that step: those who already work in practice-oriented organisations and policy bodies, outside academia.

## Notes

1  This text was presented at the fifth international conference "Medical Anthropology at Home" in Sandbjerg, Denmark. I thank the conference participants, an anonymous reviewer and Rebekah Park for their valuable comments. I also thank colleagues at home, in particular Renata Klop, Cees Smit and Maarten de Wit.

2  From its website: "Involve is a not for profit and non-partisan organisation which exists to put people at the heart of decision-making. We believe that better public participation can help solve some of the UK's most pressing challenges and lead to the genuine empowerment of people. Involve works with organisations in government, the private sector and with the community and voluntary sector to promote more and better opportunities for people to get involved with national and local decisions, services and policy making. Involve provides research, training and practical help."

3  The French speak of 'associations de malades' (associations of sick people).

4  These examples are derived from an earlier publication (Van der Geest 2007).

## Bibliography

Abma, T. and J. Broerse (2007). *Zeggenschap in wetenschap. Patiëntenparticipatie in theorie en praktijk.* Den Haag: Uitgeverij Lemma.

Abma, T. et al. (2006). Onderzoekssturing door patiëntenverenigingen. Over de waarde van een stappenplan voor onderzoekssturing door cliëntenorganisaties. *Medische Antropologie* 18 (1): 213-232.

Bleek, W. (1987). Lying informants: A fieldwork experience from Ghana. *Population & Development Review* 13 (2): 314-322.

Blume, S. and G. Catshoek. (2001). *Patiëntenperspectief in onderzoek: Mogelijke strategieën.* Utrecht: PatiëntenPraktijk.

Blume, S. and G. Catshoek. (2003). De patiënt als medeonderzoeker: Van vraaggestuurde zorg naar vraaggestuurd onderzoek. *Medische Antropologie* 15 (1): 183-204.

BMJ. (2003). *The patient.* Theme issue *British Medical Journal,* June 14, 2003, 326 (7402).

Caron-Flinterman, F. (2005). *A new voice in science. Patient participation in decision-making in biomedical research.* PhD dissertation, Vrije Universiteit, Amsterdam.

Crapanzano, V. (1980). *Tuhami: Portrait of a Moroccan.* Chicago: University of Chicago Press.

De Wit, M. (2004). "Bemoei je met je eigen zaken!" Partnerschap in onderzoek: Een positiebepaling binnen de reumatologie. *Medische Antropologie* 16 (1): 21-33.

Duyvendak, J.W. and T. Nederland. (2007). New frontiers for identity politics? The potential and pitfalls of patient and civic identity in the Dutch patients' health movement. *Research in Social Movements, Conflicts and Change* 27: 261-281.

Estroff, S. (1995). Whose story is it anyway? Authority, voice and responsibility in narratives of chronic illness. In: S.K. Toombs et al. (eds.), *Chronic illness. From experience to policy.* Bloomington: Indiana Press, 77-104.

Fischer, M.M.J. (1986). Ethnicity and the Post-Modern arts of memory. In: J. Clifford and G.E. Marcus (eds), *Writing culture: The poetics and politics of ethnography.* Berkeley: University of California Press, 194-233.

Frank, A. (1995). *The wounded storyteller: Body, illness and ethics.* Chicago: University of Chicago Press.

Frank, A. (2001). Can we research suffering? *Qualitative Health Research* 11 (3): 353-62.

Geertz, C. (1973a). *The interpretation of cultures.* New York: Basic Books.

Geertz, C. (1973b). Deep play: Notes on the Balinese cockfight. In: Geertz 1973a: 421-453.

Hine, C. (2007). Multi-sited ethnography as a middle range methodology for contemporary STS. *Science, Technology, & Human Values* 32 (6): 652-671.

Holmes, D.R. (1993). Illicit discourse. In: G.E. Marcus (ed.), *Perilous states: Conversations, on culture, politics and nation.* Chicago: University of Chicago Press, 255-281.

Kleinman, A. (2006). *What really matters. Living a moral life amidst uncertainty and danger.* Oxford: Oxford University Press.

Kleinman, A. and J. Kleinman (1991). Suffering and its professional transformation: Towards an ethnography of interpersonal experience. *Culture, Medicine & Psychiatry* 15 (3): 275-302.

Klop, R. et al. (2004). Patiënten doen mee bij ZonMw. *Medische Antropologie* 16 (1): 8-19.

Marcus, G. E. (1997). The uses of complicity in the changing mise-en-scène of anthropological fieldwork. *Representations* 59: 85-108.

Marcus, G. E. (1998). *Ethnography through thick and thin.* Princeton: Princeton University Press.

Marcus, G.M. (1999). Critical anthropology now: An introduction. In: G.E. Marcus (ed.), *Critical anthropology now: Unexpected contexts, shifting constituencies, changing agendas.* Santa Fe: School of American Research Press, 3-28.

Murphy, R.F. (1988). *The body silent.* New York, London: W.W. Norton.

Nijhof, G. (2001). *Ziekenwerk. Een kleine sociologie van alledaags ziekenleven.* Amsterdam: Aksant.

Salamone, F. (1977). The methodological significance of the lying informant. *Anthropological Quarterly* 50 (3): 117-124.

Schrama, C. (2006). Patiëntenorganisatie in spagaat. Een onderzoek naar de verwachtingen die mensen met chronische pijn hebben van patiëntenorganisatie Pijn-Hoop. Master thesis, University of Amsterdam.

Smit, C. (2005). Overzicht van het gebruik van het patiëntenperspectief als instrument bij onderzoek en beleid. *Medische Antropologie* 17 (2): 286-295.

Smit, C. et al. (eds). (2006). *Handboek patiëntenparticipatie in wetenschappelijk onderzoek.* Den Haag: ZonMw.

Smith, R. (2003). From the editor. *British Medical Journal,* June 14, 326 (7402): 1274.

Stoller, R.J. (1988). Patients' responses to their own case reports. *Journal of the American Psychoanalytic Association* 36 (2): 371-391.

Tankink, M. and M. Vysma. (2006). The intersubjective as analytic tool in medical anthropology. *Medische Antropologie* 18 (2): 249-66.

Van der Geest, S. (2007). Is it possible to understand illness and suffering? *Medische Antropologie* 19 (1): 9-22.

Van Dongen, E. and S. Fainzang (eds.). (2005). *Lying and illness: Power and performance.* Amsterdam: Het Spinhuis.

Von Faber, M. (2004). Het deelnemersperspectief binnen de Leiden 85-plus Studie. *Medische Antropologie* 16 (1): 93-104.

Zola, I.K. (1982). *Missing pieces.* Philadelphia: Temple University Press.

Sylvie Fortin

## Chapter VII.

# Anthropology within the space of the clinic: Identity, politics and methods

## Introduction

Many challenges await medical anthropologists today. They range from the intricate relationship between applied and fundamental research to working 'with' rather than 'on' or 'for' the medical field, or negotiating our methods to the evolving setting in which we do anthropology. This paper discusses a few of these issues drawing largely from research activities in Western university hospital settings and fieldwork focused on clinical practices and urban diversity.[1] It is, in some ways, a *récit*, a personal account and perspective of medical anthropology as a science that is undergoing change, arising from the practice of anthropology within the space of the clinic. I will discuss the contexts in which this practice takes place and the issues addressed both by clinicians and the research. Objects and methods will be examined from empirical and theoretical standpoints, linking classical ethnographic approaches to a local hospital environment. In these contexts, the practice of anthropology becomes a site of epistemological and political negotiation where we constantly deviate from the norm. The relationship between medical anthropology and anthropology as a whole will be explored in the conclusion. As for the relationship between anthropology, medicine and, more broadly, interdisciplinarity, Fabian (2008) distinguishes meetings from encounters in the 'field'. The first relates to an interchangeable configuration in which $x$ meets $y$ or $y$ meets $x$, whereas the second implies a social intricate relationship, often unequal, in which 'something happens' between the anthropologist and the other person. Where are we when it comes to the medical field?

From early critics of 'biomedical' anthropology (Lock and Gordon, 1988) to more recent insights into contemporary medical anthropology (Saillant and Genest, 2006), how we embrace the coming together of different disciplines has been a topic of great concern. Whether or not we distinguish multidisciplinarity (intended to be the coming together of disciplines that share a common goal) from interdisciplinarity (which refers to a closer relationship between disciplines, giving rise to an original point of view), these polysemous notions can be perceived to refer to different 'degrees' of interconnectedness (Morin, 2003). There can be no collaboration and shared reflexive stance without this interconnectedness, while sustaining a *critical distance* (Rabinow and Marcus, 2008) as an essential component of anthropology's contribution to the health domain. In other words, working hand-in-hand with physicians, nurses and other healthcare providers in knowledge-seeking endeavours does not imply the wearing of a 'white coat'.[2] This being said, thinking of interdisciplinary relations in contemporary anthropology (and medical anthropology in this perspective is a field of choice) is mapping how our discipline is evolving in its goals, objects and methods (Saillant, 2009), whether we are doing fieldwork 'at home' or elsewhere. Marcus goes a step further: 'At present, life in anthropology departments, even in the most important ones, provides only a fractured and indirect perspective on "where the action really is"' (Robinow and Marcus, 2008: 2).

However, what is a 'clinical department' in a university hospital (and therefore a university department)? It is a place of learning and knowledge in action, as medical practice is a core feature of physician training. It is also an important research environment, predominantly biomedical, where anthropological (or social) research is perceived by most biomedical researchers to be a 'minor' field of study. Whether we should negotiate a status quo or work towards a symbolic status change,[3] will have consequences, namely on how we conduct research and our capacity to adjust our methods to this specific milieu.

This is a fascinating study setting, a field site of choice in that it reminds us of the *total social fact* of Marcel Mauss (cited by LeBlanc, 2002: 72) in which a medical institution, policies governing care and resources, biotechnologies and questions related to biomedical ethics are united. We also find a diversity of professional cultures and subcultures, classes, genders, ages, religions and ethnicities, as well as individual and group dynamics. It is *an open door to the city* (Sainsaulieu, 2003) where, on an observable level, numerous social phenomena that are at work in the wider society come together. These phenomena are often exacerbated and deepened by the particular care context. As a physician colleague suggested in regards to body piercing, adolescent somatic problems, or ethical questions elicited by new technologies, the various trends that are observed in society are found in the clinic... often as precursors. Indeed, the issues that the hospital encounters are not foreign to wider society. As Van der Geest and Kinkler (2004: 1998) affirm, 'The hospital is not an island, but an important part, if not the "capital" of the "mainland".'

## Context

In contrast to psychiatry (Young, 1997, 1982; Kirmayer, 2007; Corin and Bibeau, 1995), public health (Massé, 1995) and primary care services (including the works of LeGall and Cassan, 2008; Meintel et al., 2006; Sévigny et al., 2000), the 'society-health' connection within the hospital and highly specialised care is less frequently observed and is more recently noted in the Quebec context.[4] It is an emerging site for anthropology, as practitioners themselves acknowledge, in varying degrees, the need to incorporate (or reincorporate) social, cultural, and religious dimensions within clinical space (Alvarez, 2007, 2004).

An increasing number of clinicians acknowledge the need for in-depth reflection on the course taken by medical training and daily practice. It is mainly dominated by a 'biological approach to the individual' in which 'evidence-based data' are given as the base of state-of-the-art practice. When asked about current challenges in clinical practice, many physicians who were interviewed affirmed the existence of a dichotomy between *cure* (scientific competence, knowledge, expertise, technical skill) and *care* (attitudes, as well as personal, relational, and communicational qualities):[5]

> I find that medicine has become detached from the very idea of health, with respect to life and other daily preoccupations that can be political, economic, and social in nature. It has become something entirely separate (physician, paediatric specialist, 4 years of professional experience).[6]

And again

> You've got to understand that, when we're facing a patient, all of this 'evidence-based medicine', is just one of many chapters in our head. There's a lot more than just that. And [convincing data] supply us with ideas for specific treatments but that's all... Medicine goes a lot farther and is much more vast

than simply diagnoses and treatment [...]. [...] even in groundbreaking specialties, such as my own. We don't have an enormous need for techniques or science for the care of patients, because there are no medications, or at least not at the moment. Often [what is important] is communication, establishing confidence. (Physician, paediatric specialist, 30 years professional experience)

The patient-doctor relationship (and broader health-care team-family relationship), central to the medical act, whether called a relationship of trust or a therapeutic alliance, refers to complex dynamics where a number of structuring elements come into play and where the main agents of these dynamics are the child being cared for (in the case of paediatrics), the family unit, and the healthcare provider(s). This trust relationship either facilitates or hinders the collaboration among actors within the therapeutic process. The evolution of the illness and the patient and family response (and agreement) to treatments are closely linked to this (Haynes, 2001; Desmond and Copeland, 2000).

The transformation of patient socio-demographic profiles (linked to the diversification of the urban population) and the evolution of clinical situations (including an increase in complex pathologies[7] and technological progress) present new challenges. This context promotes reflection on medicine and calls for a multidisciplinary perspective of the clinic. Research, collaboration, knowledge transfer and translation activities allow us to think differently about the clinic. They enable us to move beyond the biomedical model by presenting the clinic as a determining point from which to take the human, social, and cultural dimensions of children and their families into account. These are dimensions that should be considered alongside other aspects of care (medication, technology, or surgery ...).

A plural perspective of the clinic is not a 'natural given'. Although hospital units and professional collaborations and team (re)organisation seem to favour a multidisciplinary approach to the health issues at hand and the planning of healthcare trajectories, the decision-making process remains, in most cases, a vertical one in which the leading physician (whether an alternating attending physician or the 'long-term' treating physician within the hospital) plays a dominant role. Although much is undertaken within hospital organisation and the medical profession[8] that would tend to bring about a more horizontal decision-making framework, the recent years of fieldwork reveal clearly that this continues to be an ideal and an exception in practice.

When thinking of multidisciplinarity, physicians more often than not refer to colleagues of different subspecialties who become 'consultants' in specific cases. In highly technologically-invested areas of university paediatric hospitals, such as intensive care, oncology, obstetrics and neonatology, health issues remain in the 'cure' domain. We often seem to be very far removed from Hippocrates' (theoretically) open approach to health in which the biological, social, cultural and environmental domains coexist (Bibeau, 2002a), even if many sustain the intricate relationships today between social sciences, biomedical sciences and the humanities. This openness to broader perspectives is welcome as long as these complementary venues are embraced by fellow physicians and more inclusive healthcare providers themselves. Sharing health issues with non-biomedical disciplines is not a 'natural given'.

## The space of the clinic

Pluralist Western societies are affected by several therapeutic traditions at the margin of biomedicine that include a diversity of knowledge about the world, the body and the illness (Van der Geest and Finkler, 2004; Bibeau, 2002b). This pluralism is due to a range of factors, including the diversification of national and ethnic origins and religious confessions associated with migratory movements and also a set of variables that are more generally associated with social differentiation (Juteau, 2003) and the establishment of group hierarchy (Simon, 1997) based on age, gender and social class. The hospital environment cannot escape this diversity. Care units are meeting places for practitioners, patients and families. The clinic (understood to be a place of care and a setting where care providers and patients interact) is a place where symptoms, diagnostics, and treatments intermingle and where multiple norms and values meet and are negotiated (Fainzang, 2006; Fortin and LeGall, 2007).

The clinic's space is a social and relational space in which norms, values and professional, social, and cultural models intersect (Fortin 2008, 2006). Within culture, there are many norms and values that can be a source of misunderstanding (Carnevale, 2005; Scheweyer et al., 2004; Turner, 2003; Marshall and Koeing, 2000). The same holds true for ethical principles that guide this practice (notably, the best interests of the child). They, also, are imbued with values and norms that are socially, culturally, and historically constituted within a given context (Jobin, 2003; Massé, 1995).

The best interests of the child are such an imbroglio of our values and what we think... of the parents' values and what they think, of how things intersect, of how we transmit our information to parents, and how they receive it. What are their expectations? The place of the physician as defender of the child is not always very clear. I find that this is one of the most difficult things that we have to go through... (Paediatrician, subspecialty, four years of professional experience)

The ethical foundations of clinical practice in a pluralist context are also questioned. The notions of individuality, the decision-making processes concerning care and choice of treatments, the notion of 'informed' consent, and the relationship of these to life and death, affect these foundations and call for a renewed view (with the contribution of anthropology, some would say), that corresponds to the contemporary diversity of our social environments (Turner, 2003; Bibeau, 2000; Massé, 2000; Fleischman et al., 2001). In the context of a highly specialised paediatric hospital, clinical space becomes a place of different perspectives of the treatment of life and end-of-life processes. In this respect, death (and birth) is certainly a culturally invested moment. Conceptions of a 'good and bad death' are many, particularly in regards to the place to die or appropriate ways of dying, including the matter of accompaniment at the end. These are recurring questions at studied hospital sites. They are often at the centre of complex interactions between the care provider and patient. New technological advances in cancer, intensive care, neonatal and obstetrics units, bring about scientific and ethical debates among professionals. These are debates within the space of the hospital that reflect questions that generally circulate within society: when should life-sustaining treatments that offer no real hope of health improvement, be halted (Carnevale and Bibeau, 2007)? The passage from curative to palliative care, the prolonging of life or what is sometimes called 'proportionate or disproportionate care' (from the point of view of both the practitioner, the child and his family), perceptions of the abandonment of treatment and the modalities of end-of-treatment practices, and the choice of one treatment over another, are stages in the therapeutic trajectory that are intermingled with ethical issues, norms and values that are woven into a broader fabric of social and cultural relationships and practices.

## Objects and methods: Attuning anthropological objects and methods to the current hospital and research contexts

When collaborating with clinicians, although interest in the object of research is generally shared within multidisciplinary teams, my ongoing studies in the space of the clinic[9] are resolutely anthropological in goals and methods (observation, semi-structured interviews, case studies, exploration of phenomena, rather than verification or negation of hypotheses) while incorporating the various forms of knowledge as part of the object itself. Anthropological approaches to knowledge and methods are limited within the hospital environment and very different from classic biomedical research protocols or even qualitative research that is driven primarily by nurses. Further, if one-to-one interviews with *open* questions can eventually be understood by ethics review boards and clinical teams, practicing extended observation (four to six months) in these settings can be a challenging endeavour. We seek to document everyday (and night) life in the chosen units, team meetings, and medical rounds, and follow different key actors in their work. In order to do so, we must negotiate consent forms with the research ethics committees, while trying to honour the core philosophy of what participant observation is all about. [10]

Research teams comprise anthropologists, physicians of various specialties, nurses, and ethicists. They become a plural world that integrates, and is enriched by, a variety of perspectives. This interdisciplinarity, while promoting reflexivity by all (including anthropologists), is also a means of accessing the very 'biomedical' units, such as intensive care, haemato-oncology, neonatology or obstetrics (and the clinic for high-risk pregnancy), where social sciences are uncommon. Access and proximity to the field are made possible, or at least facilitated, by these teams that generate participation and 'acceptance'[11] of social science within a 'highly guarded territory'. This access is also facilitated by the presence of field collaborators in the clinic. They act as 'facilitators' for research assistants and, at times, as key informants. This collaboration is a fundamental prerequisite to accessing this social environment from 'within' if anthropology is to be a 'legitimate' actor in the hospital setting. By no means, however, does this belonging eliminate the multiple steps required to 'open' the field. However, this belonging certainly facilitates relations within this bounded environment and favours access to professional spaces that are often closed-off or restricted. Apart from these entry points and the sometimes extensive networking that it entails, the research process itself (i.e., discussions, interviews and observation process, as well as the increasing number of workshops and conferences in the practice setting) help to create bridges to the worlds of our respective disciplines. This 'bottom-up' method is, without doubt, at the centre of this reflexivity.

In a workshop on the identity of the anthropologist in the clinic[12] that brought together French-speaking anthropologists, my Swiss colleague, Ilario Rossi, suggested that anthropological and medical practices share a common goal, that is, a better understanding of what it is to be human (*une meilleure compréhension de l'humain*). Certainly. Nevertheless, in contrast to clinicians, we are not practitioners. We do not intervene as actors in the space of the clinic and, as a result, have a very different posture. Is it really necessary, or even desirable, to aim for a shared paradigm?

The position of the anthropologist is always one of an outsider. This is, according to Marc Augé (2006), what defines us from a perspective of method or object. In this view, observation is pertinent in that it enables us to come closer to the other, by entering, as much as possible, into the other's reasoning. This attempt at closeness does not imply, however, an assimilation of the categories put forward by the study setting. In fact, medical anthropologists have often underlined the need to maintain a distance from the object and the questioning of local categories (Rabinow and Marcus, 2008) that, in this case, are biomedical. The political character of health and the body have also been abundantly covered (Lock, 2002), as well as biopower and the relationship between biomedical sciences and the humanities (Foucault, 2001). Frequently, our daily challenge is to incorporate these structural dimensions and power relationships within an analysis that leaves room for the local meaning. In this perspective, and from a constructivist point of view, the clinical encounter is a social encounter where sets of social issues that were historically constituted by actors and set in context come into play. It is also an encounter between individuals, one who suffers and another who, in a context of power relationships, must listen and advise …[13]

Making a diagnosis is secondary to me. For me, it's important to know how I can best help the patient [facing me] and this family. So, often I will first ask how I can help in my interview. I think that that's the main thing. Then to … keep an open interview layout throughout the consultation and [remain] attentive […] to the family because often we realise that certain questions are not asked […]. And sometimes, it's precisely that… that can modify the compliance to treatment, the acceptance of a diagnosis, the follow-up, or grasping of the problem, etc. And I think that that's the most important thing in the end. It's not that I have made X diagnoses, but how I helped those people. (Physician, paediatric specialist, 15 years of professional experience)

Anthropology remains the 'face-to-face' profession (Augé, 2006) and that of the present (including its historical context). Further, because of its interest in relational dynamics and processes (*i.e.*, the inclusive study of social links and wider relationships with the other), anthropology is also the study of culture, as a set of represented and established relationships that comprise the symbolic, intellectual, concrete, historical, and sociological dimensions through which individual and group relationships are enacted.

## A few irritants

Maintaining this posture is not always easy in an environment where 'action' prevails and where so-called 'hard' sciences and *evidenced-based approaches* are the uncontested masters. Beyond the never-ending opposition of these approaches to the production of knowledge, the modes of evaluation and generation of data in health science and social science, although pursuing similar goals, can bring us to adopt a posture or a rhythm of production at times that is detrimental to what can be considered to be 'good anthropology'. Wide-scale multi-site anthropology presents somewhat of a challenge in this regard. Methods must be developed. Efforts, trials and errors are countless. Learning to practice anthropology within a team (we are often solo actors); sharing long-term observation data among research assistants; and developing strategies to ensure equal comprehension, data collecting methods, and analytical processes are part of this challenge. In some ways, this is the price to be paid for greater leeway and growing research freedom in this very biomedical environment. This being said, we must often remind our colleagues, as well as health peer reviewers, that scientific rigor takes many forms and that the production of knowledge does not follow a single pace.

Our methods are questioned in a biomedical context, along with the ways in which a problem is posed. In addition, issues of generalisation and representativeness are regularly raised. We are always in a posture that deviates from the norm. 'Hard knowledge' is still placed in opposition to the 'soft knowledge' of social sciences. In short, we find ourselves in a hierarchy of knowledge (Rhéaume 2007) where the eternal discussion between the strength of quantitative and controlled procedures wins over an open perspective – which is our strength and allows us to discover the unexpected or to make sense of apparent disorder or incoherence.[14] This often takes time (Bibeau 2009).

## Anthropology as a site of negotiations

Beyond these specific questions related to exercising our discipline, everyday anthropological practice within a healthcare institution is also a site of epistemological and political negotiation. Some see this site as a location where identities weaken. Others may see a site of affirmation – neither limited nor unconditional affirmation – but rather, the expression of a discipline resonating with its environment, a discipline whose strength lies in its capacity to move towards the unknown, *altérité* (otherness), and what animates it. However, the most prized model of health research is a research scenario in which all data or variables are identified at the outset and the study research protocol is controlled to the utmost. Here again, we deviate from the norm in a context where the 'scientificity' of the research and the medical fact is over-invested – perhaps in response to the daily uncertainty inherent in medical practice (Bourdon, 2008).

As for the weakening of identity, this may threaten newcomers who suddenly must learn to practice anthropology 'at home', to grasp what anthropological fieldwork is all about, not guided along predetermined learning trajectories as are future clinicians (which is the essence of the clinical department where every step of medical practice is marked out), but alone, on the very individual paths of their doctoral or master's research. At the same time, they must deal with the very strong professional identities of medical doctors and the nursing staff. In the care context, medical *'savoir être'* and *'savoir-faire'* make up the dominant model. This model is also highly valued in local society and research settings. In this context, one may reflect on (and question) the contribution of anthropology to the field of healthcare, in comparison to those of the 'active' professions that care, medicate, and relieve. One may also question the specificity of the discipline in investigating healthcare issues and relationships within healthcare settings, and its contribution, perspective, methods and language.

It is fascinating to see how rapidly the medical vocabulary and explanatory models invoked by clinicians become 'evidence' in papers and presentations. One must make the journey from a somewhat enraptured view of biomedicine and an unconditional incorporation of the categories put forth by clinicians to a more critical approach in order to reposition biomedicine and its tenets as *ethnomedicine* (Lock and Gordon, 1988). This fosters a more critical study of the phenomena observed. How does one carry out research in the healthcare field without borrowing a paradigm (and the language) of this field? The exercise is difficult. Some find themselves in this position, as daily negotiations drive them to (re)affirm their appreciation of their contribution. Others may tend towards a posture of intervention and care and pursue their academic training along those lines.

In short, the multi-disciplinary context, while opening to an exciting dialogue and a multiplying of perspectives on a given object, promotes this fine tuning and affirmation of identity, echoing Marc Augé (2006: 37) when he writes that *'the individual only experiences his own identity in and by its relation to others'*. In summary, boundaries are not only pertinent to thinking in terms of multi-ethnic dynamic (Barth, 1969), but also to disciplinary dynamics.

## Contemporary anthropology: A diversity of approaches and perspectives

The contributions of anthropology to the field of health are numerous, rich and diversified, from an array of theoretical stances, whether symbolic, interpretive or critical.[15] We study power relationships within the clinic, the patient-doctor and medical team relationships, professional practices, and ethical issues. We explore explanatory models of illness, symptoms, and a diversity of idioms and representations. We also examine the political dimensions of health, inequalities and social conditions that influence morbidity, power over the body, at-risk categories and norms. In short, medical anthropology has contributed to a vast and rich diversity of topics, methods, and theoretical perspectives.

## At the crossroads of applied and fundamental research

To work among, and with, clinicians is also to combine their questions and ours in order to construct research that allows us to respond to our respective and often-shared quests. With our research, we can generate knowledge that can help in the training of clinicians, allowing them to integrate various social perspectives in their practice (e.g., through clinical vignettes). We can also answer, or at least document, several practical issues pertaining to hospital life and medical practice. These concern the continuity of healthcare in specialised settings, the norms and values that guide medical decisions and requests to continue or stop treatment (quality of life, autonomy). Again, parallel or connected themes emerge that encourage reflection on the philosophy of contemporary medicine, on existential questions related to life, death, and how they are approached, on the issues and dynamics of society, and on fundamental ethical problems that transcend the borders of the hospital setting.

On the basis of this research, we can also think about the social issues beyond the phenomena being studied. As an example, the study of the clinical encounter in a context of social, cultural, and religious diversity brings us to a broader social question of the 'limits of diversity' and the search for a common ground within, and beyond, medical practice (Fortin and Laudy, 2007). More generally, a comparative approach to urban diversity and clinical practices (meaning the study of different cosmopolitan environments, such as Montreal, Toronto and Vancouver, Canada) makes room for the city as an actor in this wider perspective (Simmel, 1981). How does the city shape the clinical setting? How does this setting allow us to grasp the expression of local diversity? In this context, the emergence of a pluralist paradigm of healthcare and services gives rise to an anthropological reflection on the reconstruction of identities as a process and negotiation (Cowan et al., 2001), on the relationships between the local and the global, and on the phenomena of continuity and discontinuity between here and elsewhere (Hannerz, 1996; Marshall and Koeing, 2000). The study of different hospital settings also enables us to grasp the specificities that inform us of local and other societies beyond medical issues and the hegemony of biomedicine (Van der Geest and Finkler, 2004). From a theoretical standpoint, this comparative work provides food for thought on the intricate relationship between the micro-social and macro-social analysis, as well as a framework in which agency and structure interrelate.

## Conclusion

The clinic is a social space, a place of interaction and negotiation where a diversity of norms and values intersect (Fortin, 2008). Like society 'at large', relationships between individuals are shaped by group relationships and collective representations. In turn, these are integral parts of a given social and historical context. Added to this is the specificity of suffering and illness that, from the outset, situates actors in an asymmetrical relationship with respect to knowledge. In addition, in the migration context, these relations are (re)constructed and modulated in the process of settlement practices within the local society, family structures, and available resources (social, economic, and symbolic).

In the framework of my research, the perspective sought is often double, both inside (to grasp the universe of others, their history, and their inter- pretation, in keeping with Bibeau [2000], Kleinman [1995] or Good [1998] for example) and outside (to relocate this universe in a context that is in- tersected by locally-, globally-, and historically-constituted issues, Fassin [2000, 1996], Lock [2000a]). Like Margaret Lock (2005), I am partisan to 'just anthropology', that is, the study of phenomena related to the body, health, illness, or medicine as objects in the same way that other objects interest anthropologists. In similar fashion, S. Fainzang (2002) says that one of the challenges of contemporary anthropology is to submit biomedicine (its discourse and its practices) to critical examination like any ordinary social practice. Thus, anthropology always involves a delicate, but essential, relationship between the emic and the etic – the inside and the outside. Comparison is also a fundamental aspect of our discipline, whether in the context of an interdisciplinary or not. This comparison is a prerequisite for critical thought. This anthropology is possible 'at home'. As with all field sites, the proximity to our subject opens new windows to the understanding of our object, including the strengths and limitations of our contribution. Marcus and Rabinow (2008: 65) refer to *untimeliness* as a core feature of contemporary anthropology in a context in which disciplines and discourses overlap (and compete). This *untimeliness* favours space for the ethnographer in settings where his presence is not expected nor established.

As for our place within the field of medicine and healthcare issues, the sociologist Jacques Rhéaume (2007: 6), head of a centre for research and training in a community clinical setting, underlines how an *epistemology based on various forms of knowledge and their dialectic complementarity is the pre-condition for the interaction and social production of knowledge that undergirds the clinical posture in clinical sociology, and in the humanities and social sciences, more generally.*

Lastly, in regards to Fabian's distinction between meetings and encounters, the former would seem to be more symmetrical and the latter to evoke power relationships. However, I have had many encounters in the clinic, negotiations of knowledge and perspectives. At times, I found myself to be in the majority status, but at other times to be in the minority. It helps to understand both sides and perhaps to move towards the unknown and remain uncertain, even 'at home'.

## Notes

1   I am particularly interested in the diversity of norms and values within the space of the clinic. The fieldwork to which I refer took place in six wards (cancer, intensive care, palliative care, complex chronic pathologies, neonatal and obstetrics) in a Montreal paediatric hospital. It has now been extended to other cosmopolitan settings (Toronto and Vancouver, cancer and intensive care wards) in a comparative perspective in order to document how hospital centres in other metropolitan areas negotiate Canadian pluralism (meaning clinical practice and social relations on a daily basis) and how local urban diversity shapes the hospital environment.

2   Choosing to wear a white, pink, green or blue coat or working in 'street' clothes has bearing on the researcher's place within the clinic in relation to healthcare workers, patients and families. Bluebond-Langner (1978: 236-255) elicits this brilliantly as she shares a personal account of her initial fieldwork in a cancer ward.

3   Having peer-reviewed research grants by mainstream health funding agencies does upgrade our symbolic status in this biomedical research environment. Acknowledgement of one's contribution in this context is often closely linked to the amount of money he or she generates! And yes, this has bearing on our work. A more in-depth discussion of this issue follows.

4   The work of anthropologists Lock (2002a, 1996), Bluebond-Langner (1978), Katz (1998) contradict this, but again, I am referring more specifically to the Quebec context where much attention has been directed to community and public health and much less to the hospital context.

5   See Fortin, Bibeau, Alvarez and Laudy (2008) on this question.

6   This data comes from an ongoing study, *Clinical Hospital Practices and Urban Diversity*, funded by the Canadian Institute of Health Research (2005-2011), with S. Fortin, G. Bibeau, F. Alvarez, D. Laudy, F. Carnevale, M. Duval, F. Gauvin, and many site collaborators and research assistants.

7   By complex pathologies, I mean serious, chronic, progressive, eventually crippling and sometimes fatal illnesses.

8   The CanMEDS physician competency framework that is put forth by the Royal College of Physicians and Surgeons of Canada (Frank, 2005) specifically promotes a collaborative 'inter-professional' approach to healthcare and clinical practice.

9   These specific studies explore the themes of clinical practices and urban diversity as well as the negotiation of expert and lay knowledge in highly invested units, such as intensive care and oncology, neonatology and high risk pregnancy units, as well as in an end-of-life context.

10  See Carnevale et al. (2008) for an enlightening discussion of observation in the healthcare setting.

11  We could further discuss this need for 'acceptance' (which brings us back to a prior comment on the symbolic value of our work in the biomedical field), but, in the end, this step seems no different from those encountered in numerous field sites where we must overcome resistance and 'tame' the field in order to open doors, thoughts, and grasp what we seek to understand.

12  The workshop 'Réflexion sur l'identité… de l'anthropologie au cœur de la clinique', *Anthropologie des cultures globalisées. Terrains complexes et enjeux disciplinaires* conference, Québec, Canada, November 7-11, 2007.

13  In fact, it is worth noting that, after several years in practice, a number of physicians, confirmed specialists, have declared that listening to, and being present for the other, is now the foundation of all clinical encounters for them: 'It's more through listening that confidence is established, less in what we say' (physician, paediatric specialist, 20 years of professional experience).

14  We are reticent at times to become involved in peer review committees of large funding agencies and more widely what we often relegate to the 'administrative domain', but yet, in an environment where different disciplinary and research cultures mingle – we must reaffirm the specific character (and contribution) of anthropology to the field of health and promote the development of administrative and evaluative practices to account for it. The danger, otherwise, is to risk ending up doing 'qualitative' research that can only be distinguished from positivism by its form… Yet, if our voice is to be heard, we must find it within. After all, the biomedical setting remains a groundbreaking field for anthropology.

15  For an overview of these contributions, see Saillant and Genest, 2006; Nguyen and Peschard, 2003; Fainzang, 2002).

## Bibliography

Alvarez, F. (2007). Quo vadis: repenser la pratique médicale. In: C. Roy (ed.), *La petite histoire de Sainte-Justine 1907-2007. Pour l'amour des enfants*. Montréal: Éditions Sainte-Justine and Université de Montréal, 405-408.

Alvarez, F. (2004). Vers une nouvelle pédiatrie interculturelle. In S. De Plaen (ed.), *Soins aux enfants et pluralisme culturel*. Montréal: Éditions Hôpital Sainte-Justine, 9-12.

Augé, M. (2006). *Le métier d'anthropologue. Sens et Liberté*. Paris: Editions Galilée.

Barth, F. (1969). Introduction. In: F. Barth (ed), *Ethnic Groups and Bounderies: The Social Organization of Cultural Difference*. London: George Allen and Unwin, 9-38.

Bibeau, G. (2009). Penser notre responsabilité à l'égard du monde. In: F. Saillant (ed.), *Réinventer l'anthropologie? Les sciences de la culture à l'épreuve des globalisations*. Collections Carrefours anthropologiques. Montréal: Liber, 237-249.

Bibeau, G. (2002a). L'anthropologie: une discipline Carrefour? Débats autour de l'anthropologie médicale. In: L. Gélineau (ed.), *L'interdisciplinarité et la recherche sociale appliquée*. Université de Montréal, Université Laval, 149-160. www.fesp.umontreal.ca/sha/l'interdisciplinarité.

Bibeau, G. (2002b). Dieux étrangers, société post-religieuse et Clinique. *Prisme*, 38: 60-82.

Bibeau, G. (2000). Vers une éthique créole. *Anthropologie et sociétés*, 24 (2):129-148.

Bluebond-Langner, M. (1978). *The Private Worlds of Dying Children*. Princeton: Princeton University Press.

Bourdon, M.-C. (2008). *Regard anthropologique sur la prise en charge des symptômes médicalement inexpliqués*. Master's thesis in anthropology, Université de Montréal.

Carnevale, F. (2005). Ethnical Care of the Critically Ill Child: A Conception of 'Thick' Bioethics. *Nursing Ethics*, 12 (3): 239-252.

Carnevale, F., McDonald, M.E., Bluebond-Langner, M. and P. McKeever. (2008). Using Participant Observation in Pediatric Healthcare Settings: Ethical Challenges and Solutions. *Journal of Child Health Care*, 12: 18-32.

Carnevale, F. and G. Bibeau. (2007). Determining Which Child Will Live or Die in France: The Doctor as the Societal Moral Authority? *Anthropology & Medicine*, 14 (2): 125-137.

Corin, E. and G. Bibeau. (1995). Culturaliser l'épidémiologie psychiatrique. Les systèmes de signes, de sens et d'actions en santé mentale. In: M.-A. Tremblay, F. Trudel, P. Charest and Y. Breton (eds.), *La Construction de l'anthropologie québécoise: mélanges offerts à Marc-Adélard Tremblay*. Sainte-Foy: Presses de l'Université Laval, 105-148.

Cowan, J.K., Dembour, M.B. and R.A. Wilson (2001). *Culture and Rights. Anthropological Perspectives*. Cambridge: Cambridge University Press.

Del Vecchio, M.-J. and B. Good. (2003). Clinical Narratives and the Study of Contemporary Doctor-Patient Relationships. In: G. Albrecht, R. Fitzpatrick and S. Scrimshaw (eds.), *Social Studies in Health and Medicine*. London: Sage Publications, 243-258.

De Rudder, V., Poiret, C. and F. Vourch. (2000). *L'inégalité raciste. L'universalité républicaine à l'épreuve*. Paris: Presses Universitaires de France.

Desmond J. and L.R. Copeland (2000). *Communication with Today's Patient: Essentials to Save Time, Decrease Risk, and Increase Patient Compliance*. San Francisco: Jossey-Bass.

Duval, M., Faure, D., Lortie, A., Pasquasy, V. and G. Lapierre. (2004). Traitement des symptômes: nouveautés et défies. In: N. Humbert (ed.), *Soins palliatifs pédiatriques*. Collection Intervenir, Montréal: Hôpital Sainte-Justine, 199-258.

Fabian, J. (2008). *Cultural Encounters and Scholarly Discourses*. Conference paper. Anthropology Department, Université de Montréal, September 23, 2008.

Fainzang S. (2006). *La relation médecins-malades: information et mensonge*. Collection Ethnologies, Paris: Presses Universitaires de France.

Fainzang, S. (2002). L'anthropologie médicale dans les sociétés occidentales. Récents développements et nouvelles problématiques. *Sciences Sociales et Santé*, 19 (2): 5-27.

Fassin, D. (2000). Entre politiques du vivant et politiques de la vie. Pour une anthropologie de la santé. *Anthropologie et Sociétés*, 24 (1): 95-116.

Fassin, D. (1996). *L'espace politique de la santé*. Paris: Presses Universitaires de France.

Fleischman, A.R., Wolder Levin, B. and S.A. Meekin (2001). Bioethics in the Urban Context, *Journal of Urban Health: Bulletin of the New york Academy of Medicine*, 78 (1): 2-6.

Fortin, S. (2008). The Paediatric Clinic as Negotiated Social Space. *Anthropology & Medicine*, 15 (3): 175-187.

Fortin, S. (2006). Urban Diversity and the Space of the Clinic. Or when Medicine looks at Culture… *Medische Anthropologie*, 18 (2): 365-385.

Fortin, S., Bibeau G., Alvarez F. and D. Laudy (2008). Contemporary Medicine: Applied Human Science or Technological Enterprise? *Ethics & Medicine*, 24 (1): 41-50.

Fortin S. and D. Laudy (2007). Soins de santé et diversité culturelle: comment faire pour bien faire? In: M. Jézéquel (ed.), *L'obligation d'accommodement: quoi, comment, jusqu'où? Des outils pour tous*. Montréal: Édition Yvon Blais, 289-317.

Fortin, S. and J. Le Gall. (2007). Néonatalité et constitution des savoirs en contexte migratoire: familles et services de santé. Enjeux théoriques, perspectives anthropologiques. *Enfances, Familles, Générations*, 6, http://www.erudit.org/revue/efg/2007/v/n6/016481ar.html.

Foucault M. (2001). *Dits et écrits II, 1976-1988*. Paris: Gallimard.

Frank, J.R. (2005). *The CanMEDS 2005 Physician Competency Framework. Better Standards. Better Physicians. Better Care*. Ottawa: The Royal College of Physicians and Surgeons of Canada.

Good, B. (1998). *Comment faire de l'anthropologie médicale? Médecine, rationalité et vécu*. Paris: Institut Symthélabo.

Haynes, R.B. (2001). Improving Patient Adherence: State of the Art, With a Special Focus on Medication-Taking for Cardiovascular Disorders. In: L.E Burke et al. (eds), *Compliance in Health Care and Research*. New York: Futura Publishing, 3-21.

Hannerz, U. (1996). *Transnational Connections: Culture, People, Places*. London: Routledge.

Juteau, D. (2003). *La différenciation sociale: modèles et processus*. Montréal: Presses de l'Université de Montréal.

Jobin, G. (2003). La normativité de la bioéthique: sa structure et son développement. In: C. Hervé, B.M. Knoppers, P.A. Molinari, G. Moutel (eds.), *Éthique médicale, bioéthique et normativités*. Paris: Dalloz, 12-21.

Katz, P. (1998). *The Scalpel's Edge: The Culture of Surgeons*. Boston: Allyn and Bacon.

Kirmayer, L. (2007). The Politics of Alterity in the Clinical Encounter: Multicultural Medicine as an Arena for Building a Pluralistic Society. Conference paper *Questions in Contemporary Medicine & The Philosophy of Charles Taylor*. Montreal, Canada, October 26-27, 2007.

Kleinman, A. (1995). Anthropology of Bioethics. In: A. Kleinman. *Writing at the Margins: Discourse between Anthropology and Medicine*. Berkeley: University of California Press, 41-67.

Le Blanc, G. (2002). Le conflit des médecines. *Esprit*, 5: 71-80.

Le Gall, J. and C. Cassan. (2008). Parcours de soins d'hommes immigrants et découpage sociosanitaire du territoire: des logiques distinctes. In X. Leloup and M. Radice (eds.), *Les Nouveaux territoires de l'ethnicité*. Montréal: Presses de l'Université de Montréal, 57-72.

Lock, M. (2005). Anthropologie médicale: pistes d'avenir. In F. Saillant and S. Genest (eds.) *Anthropologie médicale: Ancrages locaux, défis globaux*. Québec: Presses de l'Université Laval, 439-467.

Lock, M. (2002). Medical Knowledge and Body Politics. In: J. MacClancy (ed.), *Exotic no More. Anthropology on the Front Lines*. Chicago: Chicago University Press, 190-208.

Lock, M. (2002a). Inventing a New Death and Making it Believable. *Anthropology & Medicine* 9, 97-115.

Lock, M. and D. Gordon (eds). (1998). *Biomedicine Examined*. Dordrecht: Kluwer Academic Publishers.

Marshall, P. A. and B.A. Koeing. (2000). Bioéthique et anthropologie. Situer le 'bien' dans la pratique médicale. *Anthropologie et sociétés*, 24 (2): 35-55.

Massé, R. (2000). Les limites d'une approche essentialiste des ethnoéthiques. Pour un relativisem éthique critique. *Anthropologie et sociétés*, 24 (2):13-32.

Massé, R. (1995). *Culture et santé publique. Les contributions de l'anthropologie à la prévention et à la promotion de la santé*. Montréal: Gaëtan Morin Éditeur.

Meintel, D., Fortin, S. and M. Cognet. (2006). On the Road and On Their Own: Home Health Care Workers in Quebec. *Gender, Place and Culture*, 13 (5): 563-580.

Morin, E. (2003). Sur l'interdisciplinarité. *L'Autre Forum*, 7 (3): 5-10.

Nguyen, V.-K. and K. Peschard. (2003). Anthropology, Inequality, and Disease: A Review. *Annual Review of Anthropology*, 32: 447-474.

Rabinow, P. and G. Marcus with J.D. Faubion and T. Rees. (2008). *Designs for an Anthropology of the Contemporary*. Durham and London: Duke University Press.

Rhéaume, J. (2007). Analyse critique de la recherche sociale dans les établissements CSSS et impacts sur l'organisation et les utilisateurs de services. Conference paper *La relation individu-société: Aspects cliniques, sociopolitiques et transculturels* conference. Montréal, November 2-3, 2007.

Rossi, I. (2003). Mondialisation et sociétés plurielles ou comment penser la relation entre santé et migration. *Médecine & Hygiène*, 59: 2039-2042.

Saillant, F. (2009). L'anthropologie au carrefour des globalisations. In: F. Saillant (ed.), Réinventer l'anthropologie? Les sciences de la culture à l'épreuve des globalisations. Collections Carrefours anthropologiques, Montréal: Liber, 2-20.

Saillant, F. and S. Genest (2006). *Medical Anthropology: Regional Perspectives and Shared Concerns*. Toronto: Wiley-Blackwell.

Sainsaulieu, I. (2003). *Le malaise des soignants: le travail sous pression à l'hôpital. Logiques sociales*. Paris: l'Harmattan.

Schweyer, F.-X., Pennec, S., Cresson, G. and F. Bouchayer (eds.). (2004). *Normes et valeurs dans le champ de la santé*. Rennes: Éditions de l'École Nationale de la Santé Publique.

Sévigny, R. and L. Tremblay (2000). L'adaptation des services de santé et des services sociaux au contexte pluriethnique. In: C. Bégin, P. Bergeron, P.-G. Forest and V. Lemieux (eds.), *Le système de santé québécois: un modèle en transformation*. Montréal: Presses de l'Université de Montréal, 77-94.

Simmel, G. (1981). *Sociologie et épistémologie*. Paris: Presses Universitaires de France.

Simon, P.J. (1997). Différenciation et hiérarchisation sociales. *Les cahiers du Ceriem*, 2: 27-52.

Taboada-Leonetti, I. (1994). Intégration et exclusion dans la société duale. Le chômeur et l'immigré. *Revue internationale d'action communautaire*, 31 (71): 93-103.

Turner, L. (2003). Bioethics in a Multicultural World: Medicine and Morality in Pluralistic Settings. *Health Care Analysis*, 11 (2): 99-117.

Van der Geest, S. and K. Finkler. (2004). Hospital Ethnography: Introduction. *Social Science & Medicine*, 59: 1995-2001.

Young, A. (1997). Suffering and the Origins of Traumatic Memory. In: A. Kleinman, V. Das and M. Lock (eds.). *Social Suffering*. Berkeley: University of California Press, 245-260.

Young, A. (1982). The Anthropologies of Illness and Sickness. *Annual Review of Anthropology*, 11: 257-285.

PART II
Medical realities
and patient strategies

Mette Bech Risør

Chapter VIII.

# Healing and recovery as a social process among patients with medically unexplained symptoms (MUS)

## Introduction

Somatic symptoms not attributable to any known conventionally defined disease have in medical classification systems been given various names such as medically unexplained symptoms (MUS), functional somatic (or physical) symptoms, somatoform symptoms or somatisation. MUS or somatisation is often used among general practitioners (GP) in Denmark where this study was made. The different terms and the use of them is currently under constant debate in medical and psychiatric research – the terminology is imbued with associations that presuppose a body and mind dualism and the medical debate concentrates on how to understand or overcome the issue of somatic versus psychiatric, as well as on establishing empirically based positive diagnostic criteria for the condition (Fink and Rosendal 2008). In this debate several studies have provided insights into how patients in primary care react, for example, towards explanations given by their GPs (Salmon et al 1999); what they choose to tell their doctors (Peters et al 2008); how they indicate what they want from their doctors (Salmon 2008); and what explanations for their symptoms they operate with (Risør 2009). Such studies point to important and heterogeneous social aspects of having diffuse symptoms that feed the discussion of medical classification with empirical data on illness behaviour, illness perceptions, daily experiences and communication dilemmas. Research on patients' lives and experiences has further focused on narratives or illness experiences of different patient groups with MUS (Bäärnhielm 2000, Cohn 1999, Dalsgaard 2005, Glenton 2003, Kirmayer 2000, Madden and Sim 2006, Nettleton et al. 2004, Nettleton et al. 2005, Nettleton 2005, Whitehead 2006). Sociological and anthropological research thus shows that patients are embedded in social processes and cultural experiences that modulate and determine their notions of being ill, their interactions with health professionals and their daily practice. This knowledge is important because it emphasises the cultural and political conditions with regard to being diagnosed with MUS and it provides the insight that patients with MUS are not a clearly defined group although they are labelled with the same diagnosis.

So far, however, most research on patients' lives has had its point of departure in clinical encounters, i.e. with an emphasis on experiences determined by health settings. Or research has been based on contacts with members from patient organisations often concentrating on retrospective experiences or narratives. Not much is known about people's health-seeking behaviour in an everyday context, living with diffuse symptoms and trying to manage daily chores at the same time as seeking recovery or healing – beyond a clinical context. On the basis of a prospective qualitative study of patients with unexplained diffuse symptoms my aim is to present an insight into the social lives and social processes of those patients and their health-seeking practices in everyday life.

## Who are the patients with MUS ?

Methodologically this study is an ethnographic study based on fieldwork data and semi-structured qualitative interviews with nine informants with unexplained symptoms. To be able to explore everyday life health-seeking and go beyond the clinical setting I still started however in general practice where informants were approached, but moved out to the homes and everyday lives of the informants immediately after having made contact. The fee for consulting a GP in Denmark is covered by the social welfare system, or, in other words, by way of one's taxes. Every citizen is attached to a specific GP who has a basic education in family medicine with individual supplementary training in, for example, cognitive therapy, communication skills or specific clinical skills. GPs are however left with poor classifications for the broad spectrum of medically unexplained symptoms and with even poorer remedies for treatment (Fink and Rosendal 2008). Accordingly, many patients are undiagnosed, GPs feel insecure about how to manage them, and they often make referrals to further assessment in specialised hospital departments. The GPs find it difficult to diagnose a patient for different reasons: They struggle with how to define the concept 'unexplained', they resist, as it were, 'making the patient ill', or they insist on looking for a well-defined disease (Hansen 2009). Patients with diffuse symptoms who consult a GP may be caught though in a fight to have their illness identified as such (Dumit 2006). They often need a diagnosis to maintain or receive social security and it is also an important step to social legitimisation among family members, working colleagues and friends.

Informants included in this study were living, respectively, in one of the larger cities in Denmark, and in a smaller provincial town. They differed greatly in age and social background, as well as in the length of time they had been suffering from diffuse and unexplained symptoms. Some were on sick leave, some were working, while others were students. As such they were situated in different phases of their lives, with different priorities and social situations. Still a general picture of strategies and illness behaviour could be derived as a result of common uncertainty, lack of legitimacy and disturbed social functions within a cultural health context that expects clear 'sick roles', symptom presentation and biomedical facts.

The informants were located in the waiting room of three different general practices during two rounds of criteria-based purposeful sampling (Patton 2007). The sampling took place over a period of one year, and interviews started during the first sampling round. During both sampling rounds only very few descriptive criteria were used: a) the patient suffers from recent physical symptoms, b) the symptoms cause him/her distress and possible impairment, and c) the patient has consulted his/her GP and has not been given an adequate or satisfactory explanation/diagnosis (this was confirmed by both patient and GP). These criteria have been used by other researchers as well (Salmon et al. 2004, Peveler et al. 1997) and have proved to be fairly applicable in family practices. Nevertheless, the sampling procedure demonstrated, that defining medically unexplained symptoms was not an easy task for the GP, as mentioned above. But the patients themselves also played a part in this definition problem. Several of the patients acknowledged the probability that their condition might be unexplained, but for different reasons not many volunteered to participate. One of the main reasons for this seemed to be the difficulty of labelling their symptoms 'unexplained' during a health-seeking process. Such a label in itself suggests marginalisation. The label seems to be useful as a working or research concept, but by definition it points in a retrospective direction: it is applied, when nothing else can be said about one's suffering. In this way it is a critical step to take to comply with having an unexplained symptom. Those, who agreed to participate in the study, seemed preoccupied with their condition, and this had already seriously influenced and brought changes into their lives.[1] However summing up, what is important at this point is that at an individual level the informants in the study agreed to having unexplained symptoms, their GPs agreed as well, but that the definition of MUS is still a medical category, being disputed and contested by medicine and not least constructed by cultural and social representations of psyche and body, positioned interactions and struggles for social legitimacy. MUS is not experienced or has the same expression for all informants, and from a medical position the designation may easily essentialise and decontextualise what is really part of their lives (Whyte 2009). The ethnographic approach however, may try to account for what fills the lives of the informants, what is at stake in their local moral worlds and how social interaction, morality and meaning make their lives significant.

The nine informants (one man and eight women, aged 31, 20, 20, 21, 22, 33, 42, 47, 58) were interviewed several times, ranging from one to five interviews with every informant, 22 interviews in total. They went through different phases of their illness during the study, and therefore the empirical data display health-seeking processes at very early explorative stages as well as health-seeking after having received a diagnosis. The interviews took place over a period of 18 months with a high concentration of interviews during the last seven months, when I was performing my second round of sampling. Semi-structured interviews were conducted for the most part in the homes of the informants, but with a few exceptions preferring the clinic (author's work place). Field study comprised interview situations, waiting rooms, and consultations with health professionals.

## The notion of healing process

The available medical classifications of unexplained symptoms often include the notion of illness behaviour or health-seeking behaviour as a defining characteristic, making implicit a dimension of 'abnormal illness behaviour' (Pilowsky 1997). The adjective 'abnormal' has now been abandoned in psychiatry and medicine, but agreement still exists that a specific illness behaviour is a defining aspect of the health-seeking behaviour for patients with MUS, however modified to a result of specific interactions between patients and health professionals (Salmon 1999). Still, substantial knowledge of health-seeking activities beyond the clinic is not provided or forms part of the notion of illness behaviour.

However, I suggest that the illness experiences and health-seeking behaviour of patients with MUS could be described as a continuous social *healing process* instead of a clinically determined abnormal illness behaviour. This suggestion is an attempt to give evidence to the impressive amount of activities and agency performed by the informants of this study at all levels of their lives and in many different situations, directed in some sense towards healing and recovery. By using the term 'healing process' I wish to emphasise that the social process and the situational and cultural context of health-seeking behaviour gives attention to active human beings who, for example, fight against – or for – categorisations, attempt to gain social legitimacy, and try to endure suffering (Kleinman 1995, Dumit 2005, Honkasalo 2009). 'Health' is then understood in a locally contingent social and moral context, and not only as a medical or biological definition referring to the absence of illness.

All illness experience may be said to imply a healing process, but what differentiates MUS from other conditions may be the dominance of, for example, a fight for social legitimacy and a concomitant notion of uncertainty which is also found in my material and which guides part of the process. In her work on the Nyole of Bunyole, Uganda, Susan R. Whyte demonstrates carefully that these people – when suffering from misfortune in life or health – try to challenge it and engage it in order to change, it rather than merely making suffering bearable (Whyte 1997). In this way her analysis shows a proliferation of action and agency in response to suffering. Secondly she shows that actions involve and influence social relations, they are acted upon and tied to social powers and institutions and have social consequences at the same time as they are closely related to, for example, physical problems. In the same vein I find Jackson (2005) and Kleinman (1995) when they write about human suffering and relate this to human existence in general: suffering is seen as 'a struggle to strike some kind of balance between being an actor and being acted upon' and 'what matters most is how one suffers and withstands it', not how to abolish suffering (Jackson 2005). Those who suffer most are those who are unable to do anything about it.

Like the Nyole the informants with unexplained symptoms in this study engage their conditions in a constant movement of actions and activities. They also engage other people and they change and modulate their situations as best they can – in order to act and to move on. The endpoint might be that health is regained but action is no warrant of success. Nonetheless, action is preferred because it signals engagement with life and ill health. This is the kind of healing process that I see taking place among those suffering from medically unexplained symptoms. Here, healing is not per definition the absence of disease, but healing covers the process of engaging with symptoms, health professionals, relatives and friends, work places, future life visions etc. in order to manage a life in distress and to create meaningful relations for one's self. Parallel to research by Johannessen (2008) the patients in this study move between different dimensions of healing – physical, social, psychical and spiritual. The healing process is not limited to pathological conditions and the cure of these, but is a hybrid transformation of body and self that builds upon associations between, for example, the social and the physical, the existential and the physical or the psychical and the physical, covering all dimensions in hybrid interrelatedness (ibid.). These dimensions are here seen and engaged with in social processes of healing within three main analytical categories: the diagnostic, the pragmatic, and the existential process.

## The diagnostic process

What I have chosen to call 'the diagnostic process' is a process not necessarily ending up with or having the intention of reaching a diagnosis. It refers to actions and interactions that have to do with a person's attempt to assess his/her suffering, to explicate it, to alleviate it, and eventually to make it disappear. It also refers to a part of the healing process, where clinical encounters of any kind play a significant role that is seeking help from professionals.

During the study nearly all informants were engaged in a diagnostic process, i.e. they consulted various experts to help them *'move on'*. Mark (31), an unskilled factory worker, for example visited his GP now and then with back pain and tiredness, but also consulted a masseur and tried spiritual healing. Hanna (social education worker, 42) consulted a chiropractor, then her GP several times with different ailments, and ultimately the rheumatologist who gave her a diagnosis – fibromyalgia. However, she continued her process of alleviation and healing by trying an electric tension module, which is primarily used for weight loss, but also had a good effect on her symptoms. She took herbal medicine for calming and consulted her clairvoyant tutor now and then. Sarah's (postal worker, 32) path during the diagnostic process was somewhat similar to Hanna's, and she also received the fibromyalgia diagnosis. Sarah was, though, very keen on exercising. Assisted by a physiotherapist she insisted on exercising, at first to make her fit in order to continue working, and later, when she was on sick leave, advised to do so by a rheumatologist. Furthermore, Sarah was one of the few informants who consulted a psychologist. This was also the case for Karen (student, 21), who was in the middle of a long assessment period, where she frequented different medical specialists and underwent various medical examinations and tests to find out why she fainted, and why she had a palpitating heart. Karen also tried acupuncture and a healing session, mainly advised by her mother. However, she did not regard this as useful.

At first sight, the reason why my informants consult, for example, a physician for advice is because of anxiety and speculations about the specific symptom, but this activity also is significant for regaining normality, being able to perform or simply being 'able' to do, what you normally do – what you do as a post worker or a factory worker, or when studying, for example, political science. Alonzo showed, that in connection with everyday life and experienced bodily signs or symptoms, the social situation of the individual determines when an illness experience requires medical advice. In such situations expectations and values concerning your role performance could influence the level of symptom containment, i.e. the degree of containing a symptom before triggering a health visit (Alonzo 1979, 1984). What is important here is that it is not necessarily the symptom or the pain itself which leads to a medical visit, but the fact that other social factors precipitate a diagnostic process. This is also the case for the persons with unexplained symptoms in this study. The norms or rules of the social situation, in which they normally find themselves – one could speak of a dominant social situation – are the primary concerns of these people. They wish to maintain their current social situation, and attempts are made to secure and restore this by consulting different health experts. Another aspect of the diagnostic process may be the fight for a diagnosis or illness (Dumit 2006), a fight which is fought against the medical or social authorities if one's illness is contested and which is often dominated by the invocation of biological/ physical facts from both sides. Such a fight was however not a prominent dimension of the diagnostic process in this context, probably because the informants were not reconciled with their health problems or they were not yet ascribing, for example, very contested conditions like CFS (Chronic Fatigue Syndrome) or MCS (Multiple Chemical Sensitivity) to themselves. I found though, that when talking about the inexplicability of their symptoms, and whether they would like to have a diagnosis, some were still hoping to find an explanation for their symptoms, while others had given up completely on doctors. But still they were engaged in the healing process, since their primary goal was to act and do something – alleviating bodily symptoms, understanding bodily mechanisms, and eventually recovering. In other words, a diagnosis could be important, but not in a strictly clinical sense. According to their social concerns it was rather circumscribed to being an 'explanation', an 'answer', or a 'hope' which could enable them to 'get on with life', as long as it was presented in a tangible way (Salmon 1999, 2007). I do not wish to claim that the patients were not hoping for a cure, because they are. But somehow cure and treatment are both closely related to the medical perception of a diagnosis. It is another context than the social one, where a diagnosis is transformed into the immediate things at stake for the patient. Hannah, who received the diagnosis fibromyalgia, was shocked and surprised by the conclusion, but at the same time also a little relieved:

> …because now I understand, why I feel like this. That it is part of it [fibromyalgia], and that it is okay to take it into account – then I do not have to get angry at myself and say: now, stop complaining.

Medical diagnoses are not necessarily useful *per se*, but they are important vehicles of the social process. They are used as proof of your suffering, a proof given by the medical system, but perhaps more important it is also proof of your attempt to do something (Glenton 2005). Whether or not you receive a diagnosis, which is rarely given when talking about MUS, the activity of consulting a physician, a chiropractor or the like is a signal to others, that something has been done. Nettleton also shows, that patients with MUS accept, that a diagnosis is difficult to make, but they still hope for ongoing medical and social support (Nettleton 2005). Support is closely related to having their symptoms acknowledged as 'genuine', which may secure an ongoing cooperation with the GP in order to help them manage their situation and perhaps alleviate their symptoms.

I see the ongoing search for support or alleviation as an extension of the sick role – social strategies for living with bodily distress lie close to identity work and they happen in a social domain 'next to' being sick. Emphasis in this healing process is put on a new life and a new kind of performance in a life with illness – not on illness without life.

## The pragmatic and everyday life process

The informants of the study experienced that their everyday lives were deeply affected by their on-going symptoms. What they experience is often a lack of energy, fatigue, pain in different parts of the body, often muscular pain, dizziness, or plain indisposition. This limits the daily functions and restricts their activities in a painstaking way. To account for this they engage in a diagnostic process which is mainly a healing of the body, but a healing process of the social everyday life is equally important. The symptoms threaten their – until now – normal performance at home, at work, and in social relations, and action must be taken to heal or re-perform this part of life in a new way. What strikes me in the field material is the overwhelming activity and strategy level concerning this social domain that point to its significance, which is at least parallel to the diagnostic process.

Lora is a young girl of 22, who suffers from a herniated disc and subsequent numbness, paralysis, and pain, which in her GP's opinion have a psychological explanation. She is disabled in many ways, but also tries to maintain a certain level of activity:

> I do get help for cleaning, but I also have to do it myself once a week. So I can do the washing together with my boyfriend. I can dust, so I do that as well, and I do most of the cooking. And I like a lot to fiddle about, so there are many, many strange things I can fiddle about with. And then, well, time flies somehow, right.

At the same time she tells me, how she has to bend down in certain ways to avoid pain, or how she has to lie down intermittently to avoid being worn out. Strategies are made, and her individual functional level is tested and accepted constantly, until '*you know what you can*'.

Mark finds it necessary to take a nap every day after work, and he cuts down on his social activities, although it is hard for him to tell his mates, that it is because of fatigue. Social functions and relations as well as physical functions are being limited and changed, when suffering from MUS. Sofia, 20 years old, who suffers from a constant headache, back-pain, and changing blood pressure, is severely restricted in her activities:

> I cannot stand up straight when I do the dishes. I end up with a severe back pain, just because I stand up for so long. It might just be 10 minutes, and

then the pain in my back is almost killing me. When I have to wash clothes, I cannot carry the laundry basket. It is too heavy. I can barely lift the shopping bags, and things like frozen food I have to leave in the corridor, and then simply sit down or lie down for 10 minutes, before I go and get them. Because it hurts. Sometimes I push myself so hard, that I have to go to bed, and it might only be 6 pm.

Despite the severe limitations she finds out, how to overcome them. Sofia talks about herself as a *'workaholic'* and forces herself to be active in other areas such as taking a course in manicure and also small jobs as a tour guide. This is painful for her, but her reason for doing it is, that 'this is something I am interested in, and I am looking very much forward to it'. Disregarding or ignoring pain is also seen in other patients. During Christmas Hannah plans, for example, to use a lot of energy on the preparations for the holiday, expecting – and planning – a collapse of her body after Christmas. In other words, she has learned how to 'postpone' total fatigue. Other informants have difficulties with their daily chores, because in addition they have children to take care of. Many activities are changed and new ways to handle things are created, such as bringing and fetching their children from the kindergarten or nursery.

Apart from domestic situations, action is also taken regarding work or study situations. Typically symptoms are neglected in the beginning, although they are experienced as very constraining. But they are overcome, they are contained while working, and then released when sleeping or resting at home. To continue working is valued and to do this Sarah consults a chiropractor and after that a physiotherapist with the explicit goal of strengthening her body so that she can perform her job. This is also part of the reason why she often suggests changes in her work routine to her boss, and in this way she can keep working, instead of taking intermittent sick leave. Karen is studying at university, and she has slowly been reducing her working hours both at the university, at home, and in different study groups. From the very beginning she plans which lectures to skip, how many hours she can spend in a study group, and, finally, how to start studying again after a break, stepping up activity level. She makes these plans not only because her symptoms demand it, but also as a kind of test, hoping, as it were, for an explanation of the symptoms, and of course also hoping for recovery. The motivation for making plans at all can be seen as a wish to do something, or to do something when nothing medically can be done – in this way her plans become part of a healing process at an everyday level.

Norma Ware has written in detail about the processes of marginalisation of CFS-patients, and many of her observations are parallel to mine, although marginalisation has just begun for the informants of my study. They do however experience role restrictions, delegitimisation, and social isolation, and they certainly try to 'remake their life worlds' (Ware 1998, 1999) in many different ways such as learning to plan with the pain or fatigue of their bodies and learning to avoid situations, where their constrained level of performance is too obvious, but at the same time to continue being active where possible. Ware argues that such marginalisation processes are dealt with in terms of resistance. I would rather argue, that what I have seen as plans, actions and strategies are part of an ongoing reflective healing process. Marginalisation is only experienced as a classificatory final result, but the remaking of a life is dealt with deliberately and conscientiously, closely connected to the framework of a life, which has been changed because of MUS symptoms, and a life that demands answers to the question: 'How do I find the best way to get on with my life?'.

## The existential process

When a disruption of your life is experienced, when bodily symptoms change your normal capacity, and you start questioning your own abilities and personal identity, it may leave you in a state of uncertainty that determines your thoughts, actions, and precautions. However, it quickly became evident from my research results that uncertainty, on the contrary, does not leave the informants passive, not even during the earliest stages of MUS. Comparing again with the Nyole in Uganda, affliction and misfortune, which also includes bodily sufferings, are dealt with through actions, engagement in the world and attempts to change it, i.e. attempts to do something about a problem: in other words to approach a problem in a pragmatic way (Whyte 1997). This is in itself an uncertain procedure, but no one actually refrains from doing something as long as all the alternatives have not been tried. The mere existence of alternatives is an important part of the approaches made by both the Nyole and the patients with MUS. There may be different solutions to their problems, and some have to be tried out. The right solution is not given from the start, and as a result uncertainty is an inherent part of this pragmatic approach. When the patients in my study seek medical care, this is just one alternative or one part of the engagement in their problems – a part which is often characterised by trying different treatments, and sometimes also by the conviction, that the solution must lie within the realm of medicine. No patient, however, stops or limits him/herself to this, suffering is always engaged. As shown above, several steps are taken within the realm of everyday life – maybe not to heal, but to alleviate and modify the suffering experienced in the realm of one's life world and social context. Notably I also see engagement in individual hopes, visions for the future, and existential choices. These are made from the very beginning as another path of alternatives, which has to be employed in the overall healing process. This part is perhaps the most important one, because it constitutes the development of new narratives, by acting and directing one's life into chosen directions (Frank 1993, Whitehead 2006, Dalsgaard 2005).

Mark, for example, believes that physical training can alleviate his back pain and tries to secure his employer's financial support in order to follow a fitness program. At the same time he hopes to get a new job in the future, but for the moment he cannot cope with the changes it will bring. Still he chooses to prioritise a long and expensive holiday, which gives him a break from the daily routine and makes him experience how he would like to feel in the future. However, being in an early stage of MUS, with only provisional sick leave, he is not only focused on the existential alternatives of his healing process. This is similar to the young student Hanna, who is suffering from stomach ache and fatigue. She feels let down by the medical system, because no explanation can be found for her symptoms. The alternative for her seems to be to start to reconsider her choice of study – did she make the right choice? She also, deliberately, chooses her own individual way of alleviation, i.e. going for walks or runs or relaxing with sweets in front of the TV.

These are just minor examples of engaging in one's existence during a time of uncertainty, but, as some of the almost chronic patients express it: 'It is equivalent to *"choosing life"* and *"knowing what you want".'* Lora, Sofia, and Sarah feel that a way to counteract their life with illness is to focus on what they are able to do on the positive and creative sides of life, while at the same time admitting that illness influences one's existence, as one pretends that it does not exist:

> You know, there are things you wish to do, for example. I also choose now and then to romp around with the kids and dance and go wild, even though I know it is not a clever thing to do. But I do it, because if I don't do it, then life sucks. So it has to do with choosing. Choose pain, or sometimes I choose to say no, because I do not want the pain – because I do not feel up to it. At other times I do feel up to it, that is, sometimes I can have pain and still be active. At other times I can have pain and do nothing – it differs from time to time. (Sarah)

Dealing with illness at an existential level is closely connected to the kind of life path one wishes to engage in, and during this process new work opportunities or educational areas may also create new alternatives to be tried out. Work is connected with ways of making a living and with social identity, which represents a dominant topic of concern for MUS patients. Former jobs can be seen as direct or indirect causes of their suffering. Others believe that their lives in general have until now taken a wrong turn, and that a new job or education should be tried out. Having a job, that is perfect for oneself, is experienced as healing and alleviating in itself. One develops one's identity and qualifications, while going through, for example, job training or education, but what is crucial here is that it is not just any job, but a job one has chosen oneself, that fits with moral existential deliberations of how to live the right life:

> Now, I have chosen political science, which is a rather ambitious study, and I could imagine that I would like to continue in that direction. But then I have, sort of, considered if it would be at the expense of my family life or such things – and then I really do not wish to carry it too far. (Karen)

Talking about personal development, some patients with MUS also frequent psychologists or spiritual supervisors in order to complement the healing process with existential aspects. They mention getting a new identity and changing their personality, while at the same time, at a psychological level, they try to shake things up that have bothered them for a long time: 'it is not only my back, but also my psyche which is distorted.'(Sarah)

As other research projects on chronic illness have shown, for example, that by Åsbring (2000, 2004), and analyses using the narrative approach by Frank, it is not rare to find patients who relate an inner meaning to their sufferings, a kind of auto-mythology (Frank 1993), where illness is the destiny that has made necessary changes in life possible. But finding advantages and meaning within suffering is also done with a flair for coincidence and an ironic attitude (Lambek and Antze 2004):

> You know, it may sound silly, but there is a meaning with it. I had to be stopped, leading the wrong life I led, where I did not take myself into consideration, and I did not use myself and my resources......so somehow it was life telling me, 'hello, you are on the wrong track', you see – so this is my chance. (Sarah)

> Then I actually think, that in a way it was a gift, that I found out, hey, you have to take care and you have to remember to keep pace with things around you. (Mona)

Significance and meaning is sought and found, and sometimes interpreted as an advantage or a gain because of one's sufferings, but always as part of an overall pragmatic healing process. Furthermore, this meaning is socially important, because it provides one with possibilities for structuring one's actions and thoughts, and it gives one a personal legitimisation of one's sufferings, when no official cause is present. Finding a meaning may also result in new illness perceptions and explanations that inform the understanding of one's suffering.

## Conclusion

The diagnostic, the pragmatic, and the existential process of healing, as illustrated above, serve to remind us that illness behaviour and illness experience can be more than just clinical encounters. Especially when talking about unexplained conditions, or conditions that are chronic or may lead to chronicity, my argument is, that when trying to understand the illness behaviour of such persons it is important to extend our approach and incorporate everyday strategies, actions, and thoughts as examples of personal healing procedures. By changing the approach we may be able to emphasise the moral reality of suffering, which is often discarded by health practitioners (Kleinman 1995). Bearing and enduring pain is a way of coming to terms with life, and the meaning with life is at stake during all three healing processes, especially perhaps during the existential process. Essentially this process expresses a moral purpose with illness, which is often overlooked in biomedical studies on MUS, representing a biomedical impossibility (ibid.). As such the healing processes contain an abundant variety of activities and reflections to counter ill health, but it is more than just clinical health-seeking behaviour, because the major part takes place beyond the context of illness, medicine, and clinical encounters, within the realm of social relations, everyday life and existential reflections.

## Notes

1   The sampling difficulties point – from a clinical perspective – towards problems with the diagnostic criteria of MUS (Creed 2006, De Gucht and Maes 2006, Kroenke 2006, Sharpe et al 2006, Sykes 2006), rather than towards limitations of the methodology of this study.

## Bibliography

Alonzo, A.A. (1979). Everyday illness behaviour: a situational approach to health status deviations. *Social Science & Medicine*, 13A: 397-404.

Alonzo, A.A. (1984). An illness behaviour paradigm: a conceptual exploration of a situational-adaptation perspective. *Social Science & Medicine*, 19(5): 499-510.

Bäärnhielm, S. (2000). Making sense of suffering: Illness meaning among somatizing Swedish women in contact with local health services. *Nordic Journal of Psychiatry*, 54 (6): 423-430.

Cohn, S. (1999). Taking time to smell the roses: accounts of people with Chronic Fatigue Syndrome and their struggle for legitimisation. *Anthropology & Medicine*, 6 (2): 195-215.

Creed, F. (2006). Can DSM-V facilitate productive research into the somatoform disorders? *Journal of Psychosomatic Research*, 60 (4): 331-334.

Dalsgaard, T. (2005). 'If only I had been in a wheelchair'. An anthropological analysis of narratives of sufferers with medically unexplained symptoms. Department of Anthropology and Ethnography, Aarhus University. Thesis/Dissertation.

De Gucht, V. and Maes, S. (2006). Explaining medically unexplained symptoms: Toward a multidimensional, theory-based approach to somatization. *Journal of Psychosomatic Research*, 60 (4): 349-352.

Fink, P., Sorensen, L., Engberg, M., Holm, M. and Munk-Jorgensen, P. (1999). Somatization in primary care. Prevalence, health care utilization, and general practitioner recognition. *Psychosomatics*, 40 (4): 330-338.

Fink, P., Rosendal, M. and Olesen, F. (2005). Classification of somatization and functional somatic symptoms in primary care. *Australian and New Zealand Journal of Psychiatry*, 39(9): 772-781.

Fink, P. and Rosendal, M. (2008). Recent developments in the understanding and management of functional somatic symptoms in primary care. *Current Opinion on Psychiatry*, 21(2): 182-188.

Frank, A.W. (1993). The Rhetoric of Self-Change: Illness Experience as Narrative. *The Sociological Quarterly*, 34 (1): 29-52.

Glenton, C. (2003). Chronic back pain sufferers – striving for the sick role. *Social Science & Medicine*, 57: 2243-2252.

Hansen, H.S. (2009). Medically unexplained symptoms in primary care – a mixed method study of diagnosis. PhD-dissertation, Faculty of Health Sciences, Aarhus University.

Honkasalo, M.-L. (2009). Grips and Ties: Agency, Uncertainty, and the Problem of Suffering in North Karelia. *Medical Anthropology Quarterly*, 23 (1): 51-69.

Jørgensen, C.K., Fink, P. and Olesen, F. (1998). Somatisering i almen lægepraksis. *Ugeskrift for Læger*, 160 (41): 5919-5923.

Johannessen, H. (2007). Helbredelse – en situeret hybrid transformation. *Tidsskrift for Forskning i Sygdom og Samfund*, Vol. 6: 57-74.

Kirmayer, L.J. (2000). Broken Narratives. Clinical Encounters and the Poetics of Illness Experience. In C. Mattingly and L. Garro (eds.), *Narrative and the Cultural Construction of Illness and Healing*: University of California Press.

Kleinman, A. (1995). *Writing at the Margin. Discourse Between Anthropology and Medicine*. Berkeley: University of California Press.

Kroenke, K. (2006). Physical symptom disorder: A simpler diagnostic category for somatization-spectrum conditions. *Journal of Psychosomatic Research*, 60 (4): 335-339.

Lambek, M. and Antze, P. (eds.) (2004). *Illness and Irony: On the Ambiguity of Suffering in Culture*. Berghahn Books.

Madden, S. and Sim, J. (2006). Creating meaning in fibromyalgia syndrome. *Social Science & Medicine*, 63 (11): 2962-2973.

Nettleton, S., O'Malley, L., Watt, I. and Duffey, P. (2004). Enigmatic Illness: Narrative of Patients who Live with Medically Unexplained Symptoms. *Social Theory & Health*, 2: 47-66.

Nettleton, S., Watt, I., O'Malley, L. and Duffey, P. (2005). Understanding the narratives of people who live with medically unexplained illness. *Patient Education and Counselling*, 56 (2): 205-210.

Nettleton, S. (2005). 'I just want permission to be ill': Towards a sociology of medically unexplained symptoms. *Social Science & Medicine*, 62 (5): 1167-78.

Patton, M.Q. (2007). *Qualitative Research & Evaluation Methods*. Thousand Oaks: SAGE Publications.

Peveler, R., Kilkenny, L. and Kinmonth, A.L. (1997). Medically unexplained physical symptoms in primary care: a comparison of self-report screening questionnaires and clinical opinion. *Journal of Psychosomatic Research*, 42 (3): 245-252.

Pilowsky, I. (1997). *Abnormal Illness Behaviour*. John Wiley & Sons.

Ring, A., Dowrick, C.F., Humphris, G.M., Davies, J. and Salmon, P. (2005). The somatising effect of clinical consultation: What patients and doctors say and do not say when patients present medically unexplained physical symptoms. *Social Science & Medicine*, 61 (7): 1505-1515.

Risør, M.B. (2009). Illness explanations and medically unexplained symptoms – different idioms for different contexts. *Health*, 13 (5): 505-521.

Rosendal, M. (2003). General Practitioners and Somatising Patients: Development and evaluation of a short-term training programme in assessment and treatment of functional disorders (PhD-Thesis). Research Unit and Department of General Practice, Faculty of Health Sciences, University of Aarhus, Denmark. Thesis/Dissertation.

Rosendal, M., Fink, P., Falkoe, E., Hansen, H.S. and Olesen, F. (2007). Improving the classification of medically unexplained symptoms in primary care. *European Journal of Psychiatry*, 21(1): 25-36.

Salmon, P., Dowrick, C., Ring, A. and Humphris, G.M. (2004). Voiced but unheard agendas: qualitative analysis of the psychosocial cues that patients with unexplained symptoms present to general practitioners. *British Journal of General Practice*, 54: 171-176.

Salmon, P. (2007). Conflict, collusion or collaboration in consultations about medically unexplained symptoms. The need for a curriculum of medical explanation. *Patient Education and Counseling*, 67 (3): 246-254.

Salmon, P., Peters, S. and Stanley, I. (1999). Patients' perceptions of medical explanations for somatisation disorders: qualitative analysis. *British Medical Journal*, 318 (7180): 372-376.

Sharpe, M., Mayou, R. and Walker, J. (2006). Bodily symptoms: New approaches to classification. *Journal of Psychosomatic Research*, 60 (4): 353-356.

Sykes, R. (2006). Somatoform disorders in DSM-IV: mental or physical disorders? *Journal of Psychosomatic Research*, 60 (4): 341-344.

Ware, N.C. (1998). Sociosomatics and illness course in chronic fatigue syndrome. *Psychosomatic Medicine*, 60(4): 394-401.

Ware, N.C. (1999). Toward a model of social course in chronic illness: the example of chronic fatigue syndrome. *Culture, Medicine & Psychiatry*, 23: 303-331.

Whitehead, L. (2006). Toward a trajectory of identity reconstruction in chronic fatigue syndrome/myalgic encephalomyelitis: a longitudinal qualitative study. *International Journal of Nursing Studies*, 43(8): 1023-1031.

Whyte, S.R. (1997). *Questioning misfortune. The pragmatics of uncertainty in eastern Uganda.* Cambridge University Press.

Åsbring, P. and Narvanen, A.L. (2004). Patient power and control: a study of women with uncertain illness trajectories. *Qualitative Health Research*, 14 (2), 226-240.

Åsbring, P. (2001). Chronic illness – a disruption in life: identity-transformation among women with chronic fatigue syndrome and fibromyalgia. *Journal of Advanced Nursing*, 34 (3): 312-319.

Helle Johannessen

Chapter IX.

# Embodiment and structures in medicine: A comparative reflection on complementary medicine for cancer in Tuscany and Denmark*

*In order to allow you to enjoy the benefits of complementary medicine, the Tuscan Health Service today provide at your disposal around fifty registered centres. With a referral from your GP and payment of the fee for specialised treatment, you may be treated by medical doctors who are experts in acupuncture, homeopathy and phytotherapy; all with full safety and tranquillity. For more information or to get the address of the ambulatory of complementary medicine closest to you, call the green number 800 556060.*[1]

In 2006 I went to the Italian region of Tuscany to gather information that would enable me to study the use of forms of medicine, other than the conventional oncological forms, among Italian cancer patients, and compare the Italian usage of these non-conventional types with those used among Danish cancer patients. A European survey had previously reported an unusually high use of 'complementary and alternative medicine' among Italian cancer patients (Molassiotis et al. 2005),[2] and it was with great interest that I wanted to learn why, and how, so many people with cancer sought other forms of treatment than those offered at the oncology clinic. Once I was there, I discovered that the political and economic structure regarding the provision of different forms of medicine differed greatly from the Danish set-up, and that Tuscan cancer patients' actions, expectations and experiences in regard to complementary forms of treatment differed markedly from that of Danish cancer patients. I also found, that the use of non-conventional medicine among the Tuscans was remarkably lower than among Danes, and thus not at all close to the high usage reported by Molassiotis et al.

In this paper, I compare and reflect upon the use of complementary medication amongst Tuscan and Danish cancer patients. Taking as my point of departure a conception of medical pluralism as a coexistence of multiple medical realities that patients move between and use for different purposes (Johannessen and Lázar, 2006), I look into the formal structures in the two localities with regard to medical pluralism, and also at patients' embodied experiences of complementary forms of medicine. The analysis suggests a close relation between the structure and the experiences of effects. The inclusion of complementary forms of medicine in the public healthcare system of Tuscany is reflected in experiences of effects as predominantly physical among Tuscan cancer patients. Danish cancer patients, on the other hand, are in close contact with a multiplicity of medical realities excluded from public healthcare, and to a large extent report on psycho-social effects.

The empirical basis of the paper was generated during fieldwork in Tuscany in 2006 and 2007, supplemented by data from several years of fieldwork in Denmark. From August to November 2006 I lived in Tuscany for the purpose of exploring the use of complementary and alternative medicine for cancer, and I returned again in April 2007 to do follow-up interviews with patients. In both localities, I have looked into the structures for the provision of non-conventional forms of medicine and interviewed practitioners advocating different forms of medicine. Further, I have interviewed cancer patients in Tuscany and Denmark regarding their strategies and experiences with a plural use of medicine; conducted a survey among Tuscan cancer patients (Johannessen et al., 2008); and had focus group discussions with Danish cancer patients in collaboration with my colleague Anita Ulrich.

## Embodiment and structures in medicine

Anthropological studies of health and sickness have always had to come to grips with an abundance of healing practices and experiences among practitioners and patients. In the 1970s the coexistence of several medical systems in one locality was recognised, and studies of medical pluralism within a healthcare system reported on differences in organisation, clinical practice and explanatory models from one medical system to another (cp. Leslie 1975, Janzen 1979, Kleinman 1980). Later the strict analytical separation into different medical systems was questioned and the lived experiences of patients using a plethora of medicines for several purposes were explored. A collection of papers from 2006 demonstrates a lively use of different forms of medicine in many countries. In this collection it is suggested that we conceptualise multiple medical realities in which patients, families and practitioners navigate as they seek to restore the health of the body and the self, although it seems difficult to point to the existence of separate medical systems in the strict sense of the term (Johannessen and Lázar, 2006). We should, however, acknowledge, that all countries have political and economic structures of medicines, and that the particular configuration of these structures differs. Within the last decades, it has become customary in the international literature to refer to 'complementary and alternative medicine' (CAM) as one category of medicine, but it is necessary to distinguish between different structures in different localities. Each country has its own pattern of therapies that are available and included or excluded from public healthcare, and it is highly relevant to look more closely at specific and local configurations in the structure of medical provisions.

From a totally other point of view, a growing body of literature on the embodiment of health and healing came forth. In a review on the anthropology of bodily practice and knowledge, Margaret Lock emphasised that the influence of subjectivity on bodily biology and social reactions to the biology cannot be ignored. She proposed that mind and body continuously metastasise into one another and that humans everywhere embody the values and norms of the society in which they live (Lock, 1993: 136-7). Embodiment as an analytical concept in medical anthropology is grounded in two theoretical approaches: the theories of bodily habitus and of the phenomenology of perception. Pierre Bourdieu was concerned that practical activity should not be constituted simply as representation and drew on the concept of habitus to point to the intimate relations between social life, enculturation and the repetition of mundane bodily practices. Maurice Merleau-Ponty's conceptualisation of the phenomenology of perception supplements Bourdieu in pointing to the body's ability to engage in the world and to build knowledge that is not formed into thoughts, but merely developed and stored in the body itself (Merleau-Ponty, 1962; Lock, 1993; Wolputte, 2004). Building on the theories of Bourdieu and Merleau-Ponty, Thomas Csordas (1994) has proposed that we conceptualise the body as a way of being-in-the-world, as a nexus for encounters between biology, consciousness and culture. The processes and practises that connect the different dimensions of the body, the embodiment, Csordas suggests to be the existential ground of culture and self (Csordas, 1994: 2ff). Since the early 1990s, the concept of embodiment has recurred in anthropological studies of health and healing for different purposes and with slightly different implications. An important contribution was given by Margaret Lock who developed the idea of embodiment into a conceptualisation of local biologies; a conceptualisation that radically questions the universal bodily biology anticipated within biomedicine in pointing to empirical evidence that not only subjective reactions to bodily disturbance differ between cultures, but also bodily disturbances themselves differ and revolve in close interplay with local cultures (Lock, 2001).

The present analysis of cancer patients' engagement in medical pluralism in Tuscany and Denmark builds on both of the above theoretical approaches. Through investigations of the plurality implied in structures of medicine and the embodied experiences of cancer patients that use several forms of medicine in the two localities, relations between medical structures and embodied experiences are explored. The fundamental question to be explored is whether patients in both local worlds alternate between multiple medical realities when they simultaneously attend treatments at oncology wards and use treatment that they find outside oncology.

## Alternative treatment in Denmark

In Denmark we find – as in many other Western countries – a multitude of diverse practitioners of medicine within and outside of the public healthcare system. The Danish Health Law states that anybody can be established as a therapist and treat sick people, provided they refrain from using specific techniques that only authorised medical personnel may use, i.e. surgery, radiation and anaesthesia (Sundhedsloven, 2007). This liberal legislation has resulted in an abundance of persons that practice what is locally called 'alternative treatment' without formally acknowledged training and authorisation. A recent survey among members of the largest associations of practitioners of alternative treatments found that among the 2,700 respondents only 2 % were medical doctors, dentists or veterinarians, 13 % nurses, 3 % physiotherapists or occupational therapists, and 7 % health auxiliaries. Three quarters of practitioners of alternative treatment modalities in Denmark have no officially sanctioned health education (Jeppesen et al. 2007: 23-26). The same survey estimated that although many Danes seek treatments offered outside the public healthcare system for wellness or prevention, a large number seek them for treatment of disease. This is confirmed in a nationwide, population based and representative study, in which 59 % of those who had used alternative treatment modalities did so because of a disease (Lønroth and Ekholm, 2006).

Some forms of medicine that are elsewhere excluded from public healthcare have recently been included in the Danish public healthcare system. Since 2001, acupuncture has been partly reimbursable if provided by a medical doctor in the treatment of pain or rheumatism, and some hospital departments have included acupuncture and visualisation for pain treatment. These initiatives have, however, passed without any change in the official status of the treatment modalities.

Most Danes suffering from cancer receive biomedical treatments, but a substantial number complement this with other treatment modalities. Surveys estimate that between 36 % and 75 % of Danish cancer patients have a plural use of medicines, the mostly used non-biomedical forms being natural medicine, acupuncture, reflexology and spiritual healing (Molassiotis, 2005; Anker, 2006).[3] 'Natural medicine', a local category that includes as diverse products as herbal remedies and teas, homeopathic remedies, shark cartilage, Coenzyme Q10, and much more, is most widely used. Around half of the Danish cancer patients declare that they supplement conventional treatment with natural medicines, with the aim of counteracting adverse effects of chemo and radiation therapy or to stimulate the immune system. The natural remedies are mostly recommended by family and friends and bought in chemists' shops, health shops or supermarkets (Anker, 2006: 25-28).

Mental and emotional issues also seem to be important in Danish cancer patients' use of alternative treatment modalities. Around 25 % have practiced some kind of mental technique after they received the cancer diagnosis, most commonly relaxation (17 %), visualisation (12 %) and meditation (10 %). A minority of 5-10 % have consulted what is in Danish called a 'healer' (Damkier, 2000; Anker, 2006) – a heterogeneous category of persons practicing spiritual healing, some forms of massage, prayer, the laying on of hands, etc. In a focus group with cancer patients, a woman said that she consulted a 'healer' in order 'to get peace of mind', and that she had done this continuously since she had breast surgery four years ago. This woman, as many other Danish cancer patients, experienced alternative treatment modalities as useful for the provision of mental and emotional support, and she found this imperative to stand the physical and emotional hardships of cancer and conventional cancer treatment, as well as for the prevention of relapse.

Danish cancer patients most often consult non-medical practitioners when they seek professional complementary help, and in general they do not discuss these matters with the oncologists. Those that had tried to discuss the use of complementary approaches with their oncologists, most often experienced that the oncologists found it a waste of money and of no use. The patients therefore in general avoid discussing these matters with the medical doctors, but keep on using alternative treatment on their own.

Although the patients hope that the alternative approaches may help them to become well, they repeatedly distinguish between the curative competences of the medical doctors and the general supportive competences of alternative treatments.

## Non-conventional and complementary medicine in Tuscany

In Tuscany, as in all other regions of Italy, medical doctors have a monopoly in the treatment of disease, which means that the variety and number of non-medical practitioners here is much smaller than in Denmark. It is possible to find reflexologists, practitioners of reiki, or other non-medical practitioners, but they restrict their work to the improvement of well-being (*benessere*). A number of medical doctors and medical clinics do, however, offer forms of treatment that in the international literature is classified as CAM. Normally these forms of medicine are called 'non-conventional medicine' in the local vernacular (*medicine non convenzionali*) (MnC), and some of these have recently been included in the public healthcare system. In Italy, each of the 20 regions of the country has the right and obligation to establish regional regulations of healthcare within the frames of that which, at the national level, have been formulated as basic services (*Livelli Essenziali di Assistenza*). Today, acupuncture, herbal medicine and homeopathy are included in public healthcare in Tuscany, and the region is recognised by the EU and WHO as a front region regarding inclusion of complementary forms of medicine.

Since the first opening towards traditional Chinese medicine in 1987 the regional health plans of Tuscany have increasingly included MnC, and the Regional Health Plan of 1999-2001 is considered the definitive breakthrough for official recognition of the field as it established a committee with the aim of initiating investigations of non-conventional medicines. The initial explorations were followed by regional support projects on development and exploration of a wide variety of non-conventional medicines within the public healthcare system during 2002-2004, but in the health plan of 2005-2008 the regional interest in MnC was narrowed down to four kinds of medicine: acupuncture/TCM, homeopathy, phytotherapy and manual medicine. These four treatment modalities became reimbursable within public healthcare and three reference centres (on TCM, homeopathy and phytotherapy) were established. In 2007 the process of selection and inclusion of CAM seemed to conclude however, as the regional council legislatively established acupuncture, homeopathy and phytotherapy as basic health services to be provided by the public healthcare system of Tuscany. On the homepage of the regional health authorities these are now designated as 'complementary medicines' and one finds introductions to the treatment modalities, their areas of competence, information and links to the three reference centres, and a list of 57 medical clinics that provide complementary medicines within the public healthcare system of Tuscany.

The Tuscan cancer patients that participated in the present project were identified at two out-patient oncology clinics. A questionnaire survey on their use/non-use of different forms of medicine revealed that they were modest users of complementary medicine, as only 17 % of the respondents reported to have used some complementarities after the cancer diagnosis. The most common complementary modalities were herbal medicine (used by 52 % of all those who used some complementary medicine), homeo-pathy (used by 30 %) and acupuncture (used by 13 %) (Johannessen et al., 2008). This pattern in use corresponds very well with earlier studies of complementary medicine use among Tuscan cancer patients (Crocetti et al., 1998). Cancer patients' preferences for these forms of treatment correspond well with the Tuscan inclusion of exactly these three forms of medicine in the public healthcare system. It is, however, quite interesting to note that only a few of the cancer patients that we talked with had ever heard about the regional policy in this area. Conversations with doctors and nurses at oncology departments revealed that doctors never introduced patients in curative chemotherapy to any forms of complementary medicine, and that they in general were quite sceptical about the relevance of these forms of medicine for cancer. Especially herbal medicine was questioned due to po-tential counter-effects to chemotherapy, while the belief in the potency of homeopathy and acupuncture was low in comparison with ordinary drugs.

The widespread use of herbal medicine among the Tuscan patients pre-dominantly consisted in the use of Aloe that they bought at local herbal shops (*erboristerie*) without consulting a medical specialist. Many patients reported that they had been advised by family or friends to use Aloe as a liquid mixed with liquor (*grappa*) and honey to strengthen the body and to enhance physical wellbeing in general. Only one patient reported to have been in touch with the regional reference centre for phytotherapy, and she said that she never took the herbal medicine she acquired with the aim of stimulating her immune system, because her oncologist advised her against it, due to fear that it would counter-effect the chemo.

Users of homeopathy and acupuncture found the providers through recommendations from their social network or from the Internet. The reasons to try these complementary medicines were most often to increase the body's ability to fight the disease or to increase physical wellbeing. Common explanations among those that did not use complementary medicine in connection with their cancer were that they were satisfied with the conventional treatment, that their doctor had never recommended it, and that they did not find non-conventional medicine suitable for serious diseases like cancer, while it might be useful in less serious instances.

## Structures and medical realities

When considering the structures in medical provision, it seems that Denmark and Tuscany represent two different versions of medical pluralism, two versions that in some way represent the extremes in the international landscape of configurations.

In Denmark a large part of the treatments available for cancer patients are structurally positioned as alternatives to biomedicine. Very few medical doctors engage in alternative practices and only a few (acupuncture and visualisation) are included in the public healthcare system as auxiliaries for pain management. Simultaneously, a large number of alternative treatment modalities are available and legally accepted outside the public healthcare system. What appears is an overall healthcare system with a clear division between biomedical treatments offered by medical doctors within the public healthcare system, and an alternative healthcare sector comprising a highly heterodox group of non-medical practitioners that provide a variety of unregulated alternative forms of treatment outside the public healthcare system. This situation provides an overall division into two very different medical realities that patients and providers may engage in, and as the alternative sector is uncontrolled and comprises a vast number of different kinds of therapies, the number of medical realities available is vast.

In Tuscany the configurations are different. In this locality only medical doctors are legally allowed to treat sick persons, but contrary to the Danish situation a substantial number of medical doctors provide those kinds of treatment that in Denmark are provided by non-medics. Three of these (homeopathy, herbal medicine and acupuncture) are by now formally included as basic services within the public healthcare system. It seems difficult to talk about different medical realities in Tuscany as no real alternatives exist. The biomedical reality is dominant and the basic premises of this system are not challenged, so to speak. On the home page of the Tuscan Health Services, complementary medicine is indicated as relevant for minor health problems that are more or less chronic, e.g. sleeplessness, digestive problems and allergies. But not only the kind of problems for which complementary medicine is considered relevant, supports the hegemony of biomedicine. Also the way the effects of complementary medicines are envisioned demonstrates biomedical hegemony. An example is from a clinic that administrates Bach's flower remedies. These remedies are originally supposed to relieve emotional problems such as loneliness, fear, lack of interest in the present, etc.[4] But the use of Bach's flower remedies in the Tuscan clinic revealed that the medical doctor administrating them attributed physical effects to them, as she mentioned that the remedies could counter effect issues such as inflammation, pain and hot flushes. This example very clearly demonstrates how a technique that originally was referring to issues normally excluded from the realm of biomedicine has been reformulated within a biomedical frame of understanding. The medical doctor that administrated Bach's flower remedies did not consider these relevant for cancer patients. Likewise, conversations with medical doctors at the reference clinics for traditional Chinese medicine and for herbal medicine in Tuscany, revealed that they did not consider their treatments as relevant for cancer patients, except for the potential of alleviating side-effects such a pain and nausea.

Studies from other countries demonstrate structures of healthcare that differ from the Danish and the Tuscan situation. In the UK, for example, one finds medical doctors that provide complementary methods at hospitals and other clinics within the public healthcare system, and a number of non-medical practitioners outside the public healthcare system (Cant and Sharma, 1999). Similar mixed patterns are found in the USA and in Germany, China, Japan, Pakistan and Australia, to mention just a few, with local variations of the organisation of the co-existence, collaboration and funding (Baer, 2004; Maretzki and Seidler, 1985; Unschuld, 1998; Ohnuki-Tierney, 1984; Tovey et al. 2007). In consideration of the international situation, Denmark and Tuscany become examples of two radical systems of healthcare. In Denmark we find two separate categories of healthcare, a biomedical and an alternative, of which the latter is highly heterogeneous. This gives patients the potential to engage in and to combine many different medical realities according to personal preferences and finances. In Tuscany we find one overall medical reality including a limited number of complementary offers that have been 'tamed' or aligned to biomedicine in terms of what they can be used for (minor, chronic physical problems) and what they can accomplish (physical relief for problems that cannot be cured with biomedical approaches).

## Embodying medical structures

To understand the differences between the use and experience of complementary treatments as reported by the Tuscan and the Danish cancer patients, I propose the concept of embodiment as relevant. The concept of embodiment implies a certain indeterminacy in the sense that the world – and the body itself – is something that is objectified by a subject according to values and traditions in the cultural environment in which a person lives (Csordas, 1990: 38-39). In our bodily being in the world, we act and react to the world in modes that are at our disposal in the cultural milieu in which we live, and we sense our bodies in ways that are influenced by the cultural schemes available to us in the localities in which we live. This implies that bodies can be approached as situated agents that embody their context as they articulate and act on behalf of sensations from within as well as from the outside. In extension of Csordas' proposition, it becomes clear that cancer patients in Tuscany and Denmark embody their contexts and sense the effects of complementary forms of medicine in accordance with the cultural milieu in which they live.

The Tuscan cancer patients are very observant to the physical manifestations of their body and they seek complementary forms of medicine that may ease physical discomfort, e.g. nausea and tiredness, or enhance physical processes such as digestion or immune response. Those that consult practitioners of complementary forms of medicine, usually seek medical doctors that provide homeopathy or acupuncture. But even if the patients do not consult a practitioner, but buy Aloe or other herbal products in the herbal shops, they predominantly expect and experience the medicines to counter-affect the physical side-effects of the disease and the biomedical treatment. Among the 132 Tuscan cancer patients we met, hardly anyone talked about psychological causes of cancer, or of the need to work with psychological aspects as part of their treatment. Only one patient, a man in his forties, used some kind of psychological treatment, as he consulted non-medical practitioners of Emotional Freeing Therapy and Reiki. He himself believed that he was aware of these forms of therapy because his wife is a foreigner. According to him, Italians in general only think about medical doctors as relevant for treatments. He sought the complementary therapies as a means to help him relax during the hardships experienced with the diagnosis and the biomedical treatment, as a psychological support to stand the hard conventional treatment. On being questioned by me, he denied that his use of these therapies had anything to do with a supposition of mental causes of the disease or a need for mental support for recovery from the cancer.

According to a study of the medical pluralism in Emilia-Romagna, the region just north of Tuscany, people in this region tend to blend ideas from modern biomedicine with ideas from the traditional humoural medical system (Whitaker, 2003). In this mixed view of disease and medicine – that, according to Whitaker, is shared by patients and medical doctors – focus is on physical issues such as heat and microbes, and treatments considered relevant are predominantly physical, although they may be non-conventional. Whitaker claims, that a particular blend of modern biomedicine and ancient humoural medicine lies behind the rapid acceptance of acupuncture and the prevailing use of spas for the treatment of diseases (Whitaker 2003: 361-62). Likewise, the strategies of cancer patients in Tuscany, and the prevailing insistence on the physical aspects of disease and therapies, may be connected to a survival of humoural ideas in the health care of contemporary Italy.

Danish cancer patients also use complementary treatment modalities to counter-effect nausea and tiredness and to improve digestion and the immune response. But at the same time an articulation of the psychological aspects related to the cancer is quite common among the Danish patients, and the idea that it is necessary to complement the biomedical treatment with therapies that can contribute to healing of the mental and the emotional is common. In a study on Danish cancer patients' attendance with practitioners who provided energy healing, Majken Belusa found that patients substantiated their use of these therapies on a need to meet existential issues, a wish for caring, and as an aid to tackle psychological issues related to suffering from cancer, to understand ones situation and to find peace in a spiritual understanding of the situation (Belusa, 2009). Danish cancer patients seem to put emphasis on the disease as a phenomena interlocking with several different aspects of life – with several 'realities' – and they tend to seek different kinds of practitioners that each contribute to a common whole: the medical doctor to fight the abnormal cancer cells, the healer to get a hold on existential issues, the reflexologist to support the general functioning of the body, etc.

In the conception of multiple aspects as relevant for the curing and caring of disease, the Danish patients are in line with patients in many other countries where non-medical practitioners are allowed to administrate complementary therapies. In Australia, for example, doctors seem to be as hesitant in support of complementary medicine for cancer as the Danish and Italian doctors (Broom and Adams, 2009); but Australian cancer patients use complementary medicines as a means to enhance their control of the situation, to retain a sense of power within disease and treatment processes, and to gain inner peace and relaxation, and they consider these issues not as a means of coping, but as integral parts of a multidimensional healing process (Broom, 2009: 78-79).

A holistic approach to cancer and other diseases is most often considered as positive by social researchers that look into complementary forms of medicine (cp. Broom and Tovey, 2008). A report from the European Society of Mastology likewise acknowledged the relevance to meet the emotional and spiritual needs of the cancer patients, and complementary medicine was considered potentially relevant in this respect although the authors also pointed to priests and psychologists as important contributors of aid (Baum et al., 2006). But in a critical perspective, the holistic approach to disease and healing can be conceptualised as 'holistic sickening' contributing to overwhelming implications of the disease (Sered and Agigian, 2008). Although patients often voice a positive notion of the holistic approach to cancer in one-time interviews, studies that follow patients for prolonged periods of time have shown that over time they falter in their acceptance of the multidimensional aspects of the disease and treatment and in their ability to follow the different advice they receive of what to do (Broom and Tovey, 2008; Belusa, 2009).

The differences in the prevailing tendencies among Tuscan and Danish cancer patients' experiences and actions in regard to complementary treatments seem to be examples of the embodiment of culture and self. The Tuscans embody complementary medicine as a means to enhance physical issues related to the disease and the biomedical treatment. So do the Danish cancer patients, but at the same time they embody a subjective experience of psycho-social issues as important for the onset of the disease and for its healing, as well as for the capability to live with the disease and the biomedical treatment. One could extrapolate these findings in support of Margaret Lock's idea of local biologies. Just as Lock found differences in American and Japanese women's physical sensations of the menopause (Lock, 2001), the Danish and Tuscan cancer patients demonstrate differences in what kinds of effects they expect and experience from complementary medicines. It seems like the patients from these two different structures of medical provision seek and experience different types of effects from treatment modalities that in theory should be the same.

## Multiple medical realities revisited

The comparison of medical plurality in Tuscany and Denmark demonstrates affinities between institutional structures, experience, and practice in the two localities. In Tuscany, medical doctors are granted the monopoly on the treatment of diseases and practise the forms of non-conventional medicines that have recently been included in the public healthcare system. The Tuscan cancer patients predominantly use the very same kinds of medicine although most were unaware of the policy and did not receive complementary treatments within the public healthcare structure. Tuscan patients expressed general confidence in the competences of medical doctors, also regarding non-conventional forms of treatment, and they predominantly expected and experienced effects that referred to the biological body and physical features. This points to a hegemonic position of biomedicine. Medical doctors were recognised as competent in regard to complementary forms of medicine, and the patients seemed to be content with medical paradigms of biological and physiological aspects of the body. The patients recognised the need for emotional support but did not consider this a matter of treatment and this aspect therefore cannot be considered as part of a medical reality.

In contrast to this, the Danish configuration in medical plurality is characterised by a division between conventional and alternative treatment modalities in policy and discourse, as well as in the practice of patients and practitioners. In the Danish case, an exclusive but tolerant policy regarding alternative treatment modalities is closely tied to the fact that very few Danish doctors affiliate with alternative organisations. Alternative treatment modalities are nested in the practice of non-medical practitioners outside the public healthcare system, and the patients readily accept and acknowledge the competences of these alternative practitioners to be different than the competences of medical doctors. The Danes seek cure of the cancer in the public healthcare system and support of the body as a physical, emotional and spiritual feature through alternative forms of medicine on a private market, and they rarely discuss these matters with the medical doctors. The division is present in expectations and experiences of effects, and the Danes engage in medical realities that differ more profoundly than the ones Tuscans engage in, as the medical realms span from a purely conventional biomedical realm focussed on combating the disease, to complementary medical realms focussed on supporting the body in biological as well as spiritual and emotional terms.

## Notes

\* The project was supported by the University of Southern Denmark, Centro per lo Studio e la prevenzione oncologica (Florence), and the Danish Research and Knowledge Center of Alternative Medicine. I thank Elisa Pasquarelli, University of Perugia, for assistance during fieldwork in Italy, and Anita Ulrich and Majken Belusa, University of Southern Denmark, for collaboration and discussions on comparative perspectives on the plural use of medicines for cancer.

1 Homepage of the Tuscan public health authorities, retrieved 27th of December, 2007, from (http://www.salute.toscana.it/campagne/campagna_medicine_complementari. shtml) (my translation).

2 According to this survey, Italian cancer patients had the highest use of complementary medicines (CAM) in Europe as 73 % had used some kind of CAM, whereas 36 % of Danish cancer patients use CAM (close to the European average), and the Greeks were at the bottom with only 14 % of cancer patients using CAM (Molassiotis 2005).

3 According to Anker (2006), 54 % of the cancer patients that called the support-line of the Danish Cancer Society used some kind of natural medicine since the onset of cancer. 37 % have consulted a practitioner of alternative treatment modalities. Most commonly consulted practitioners were acupuncturist (consulted by 20 %), reflexologists (14 %) and spiritual healers (10 %).

4 http://www.bachcentre.com/centre/remedies.htm, retrieved June 19, 2009.

## Bibliography

Anker, N. (2006). *Kræftpatienters brug af alternativ behandling. En undersøgelse blandt brugerne af Kræftens Bekæmpelses telefonrådgivning.* Kræftlinien, Copenhagen: Kræftens Bekæmpelse.

Baer, H. (2004). *Toward an Integrative Medicine – Merging Alternative Therapies with Biomedicine.* Walnut Creek: AltaMira Press.

Belusa, M. (2009). Det gode liv – lykkes det? Kræftpatienters oplevelser hos behandlere der arbejder med healing. PhD-dissertation. Faculty of Health Sciences, University of Southern Denmark.

Broom, A. (2009). 'I'd forgotten about me in all of this'. Discourses of self-healing, positivity and vulnerability in cancer patients' experiences of complementary and alternative medicine. *Journal of Sociology*, 45 (1): 71-87.

Broom, A. and Adams, J. (2009). Oncology clinicians' accounts of discussing complementary and alternative medicine with their patients. *Health*, 13 (3): 317-36.

Broom, A. and Tovey, P. (2008). Exploring the Temporal Dimension in Cancer Patients' Experiences of Nonbiomedical Therapeutics. *Qualitative Health Research*, 18 (12): 1650-61.

Cant, S. and Sharma U. (1999). *A New Medical Pluralism? Alternative medicine, doctors, patients and the state.* London: Routledge.

Csordas, T. (1990). Embodiment as a Paradigm for Anthropology. *Ethos*, 18 (1): 5-47.

Csordas T. (1994). *Embodiment and Experience: The Existential Ground of Culture and Self.* Cambridge: Cambridge Studies in Medical Anthropology.

Crocetti, E., Crotti, N., Feltrin, A., Ponton, P., Geddes, M. and Buiatti, E. (1998). The Use of Complementary Therapies by Breast Cancer Patients attending Conventional Treatment. *European Journal of Cancer,* 34: 324-328.

Damkier, A. (2000). Kræftpatienters brug af alternativ behandling. PhD-dissertation. Faculty of Health Sciences, University of Southern Denmark.

Janzen, J. (1979). Pluralistic legitimation of therapy systems in contemporary Zaire. In: Ademuwagun, Z.A. (ed.), *African Therapeutic Systems.* Honolulu: Crossroads Press.

Jeppesen, S. et al. (2007). *Analyse af det danske udbud af komplementær og alternativ behandling.* Odense: CAST.

Johannessen, H. and Lázár, I. (eds). (2006). *Multiple Medical Realities – Patients and Healers in Biomedical, Alternative and Traditional Medicine.* London: Berghahn Press.

Johannessen, H., Hjelmborg, J., Pasquarelli, E., Fiorentini, G., Di Costanzo, F. and Miccinesi, G. (2008). Prevalence in the use of complementary medicine among cancer patients in Tuscany, Italy. *Tumori,* 94: 406-410.

Kleinman A. (1980). *Patients and Healers in the Context of Culture.* Berkeley: University of California Press.

Leslie C. (1975). Pluralism and integration in the Indian and Chinese medical systems. In: Kleinman, A. (ed.), *Medicine in Chinese Cultures,* U.S. Government Printing Office, Washington D.C.

Lock, M. (1993). Cultivating the Body: Anthropology and epistemologies of bodily practice and knowledge. *Annual Review of Anthropology* 22: 133-55.

Lock, M. (2001). The Tempering of Medical Anthropology: Troubling Natural Categories. *Medical Anthropology Quarterly,* 15 (4): 478-92.

Lønroth H. and Ekholm O. (2006). Alternativ behandling i Danmark – brug, brugere og årsager til brug. *Ugeskrift for Læger,* 168 (7): 682-86.

Maretzki, T.W. and Seidler, D. (1985). Biomedicine and naturopathic healing in West Germany. A Historical and ethnomedical view of a stormy relationship. *Culture, Medicine and Psychiatry,* 9: 383-421.

Merleau-Ponty, M. (1962). *Phenomenology of Perception.* London: Routledge and Keagan Paul.

Molassiotis, A. et al. (2005). Use of complementary and alternative medicine in cancer patients: a European survey. *Annals of Oncology,* 16: 655-663.

Ohnuki-Tierney, E. (1984). *Illness and Culture in Contemporary Japan. An anthropological view.* Cambridge: Cambridge University Press.

Sered S. and Agigian, A. (2008). Holistic sickening: breast cancer and the discursive worlds of complementary and alternative practitioners. *Sociology of Health & Illness,* 30 (4): 616-31.

*Sundhedsloven* (2007). Copenhagen: Danish Ministry of Health.

Tovey, P., Chatwin, J. and Broom, A. (2007). *Traditional, Complementary and Alternative Medicine and Cancer Care. An international analysis of grassroots integration.* London: Routledge.

Unschuld, P.U. (1998). *Chinese Medicine*. Paradigm Publications: Taos, New Mexico.

Whitaker, E.D. (2003). The Idea of Health: History, Medical Pluralism, and the Management of the Body in Emilia-Romagna, Italy. *Medical Anthropology Quarterly* 17 (3): 348-75.

Wolputte, S. (2004). Hang on to Your Self: Of Bodies, Embodiment, and Selves. *Annual Review of Anthropology* 22: 251-69.

Arantza Meñaca

# Chapter X.

# Biomedicine in the health pragmatics of Ecuadorian migrants[1]

Migrants are easily associated with the topic of multiple medical realities. It is generally assumed that, with immigration, the context of health care in the arrival societies becomes more diversified, more multicultural. Let me present two simplified perspectives. It can be said that the medical pluralism of their health systems is enhanced with the 'traditional' practices imported from migrants' countries of origin: experts in these 'sciences and arts' might be available not only to the 'ethnic' community, but also to the whole society (Ma, 1999; Kim *et al.*, 2002; Carvalho, 2006). From another point of view, it is well known that immigrants encounter barriers to access, and experience misunderstandings with, the official health systems in the arrival countries that can be partially interpreted as related to different pragmatics and ways of understanding health care (LaVeist, 2005).

In these pages, the approach taken is closer to the second perspective. The focus is not on the co-existence of different healing alternatives and migrants' contributions to this complex arena. Following Els van Dongen (2008), multiple medical realities are instead defined as the different lines of thought used to construct and understand health, disease, and care. I want to centre in the 'selective and affinitive organising principles' (Burke, 2007) that frame people's health seeking processes, attitudes and opinions related to health and the medical resources available. Note that I have spoken of 'people' and not of 'migrants' as, in my experience, there are basic shared ideas in medical anthropology that cannot be taken for granted when talking about migrants (Meñaca, 2007a). One of them is that the multiplicity of medical realities is not only related to ethnicity or country of birth: age, sex, profession, socio-economic status, religion, neighbourhood, etc. are other factors involved in defining our cultural positions. Moreover, multiple medical realities are not only found when studying the general population, as within biomedicine itself, different logics can also be found: ways of constructing the body, diseases and health depending on professions, specialisms, services, policies, health structures, institutions, etc. (Hahn and Kleinman, 1983; Comelles, 2004).

Given this general framework, there is one characteristic in our contemporary world to which migration draws attention: the knowledge and use of a variety of medical resources allocated in different countries (Kangas, 2002). Transnational migrant families' health seeking processes involve providers both in the countries of origin and arrival, which increases the diversity of their health care practices (Tiilikainen, 2006). In the transnational medical itineraries of Ecuadorian migrant families, as we will see, a central space is occupied by the biomedical resources of both the countries of origin and arrival. Biomedicine will, therefore, be the focus of this article. Its aim is to show how the conflictive relationship between the Spanish health care system and Ecuadorian migrants is not based on totally different ways of understanding health and biomedicine, but on the networks and resources that migrants mobilise to solve their health problems while sharing the core principles of biomedicine's self-definition and logic.

Ecuadorian and Spanish health care systems characterise the context where health care seeking practices take place. Both in Ecuador and in Spain, biomedicine is the *hegemonic medical model* (Menéndez, 2005) and biomedical providers are the most frequently used resource. The main difference between the two countries is the availability of a free health care system. In Spain, access to most primary health care and hospital services is free and universal, dental care being the main exception. All migrants registered in the municipality – no permit of residence is needed – have access to the system. 13.5 % of the population, mainly those of higher socio-economic status, has additional private insurance (González, Urbanos and Ortega, 2004). It is different in Ecuador, where public health insurance covers only 19 % of the population and, in migrants' opinion, most of the time it lacks the necessary resources to give proper attention. The Ministry of Health and some Municipalities provide different primary health care programmes free of charge and other resources, including hospital technologies, at low cost. However, these programmes and others offered by different NGOs are not enough: in Ecuador 40 % of the health care costs are paid directly by the families (O.P.S., 2001). A very small part of this is used to contract private medical insurance, while the majority is spent on direct services of consultation and pharmacy.

Biomedicine is central to this article and also to the health care practices of the Ecuadorian migrants I have worked with. It does not mean that there is no use for 'traditional' and complementary medicines (CAM), but that both in Ecuador and with migration, they have a subaltern place.[2] Ecuadorian migrant families have not increased, at least in the first five years, their repertoire of CAM used on an everyday basis. More over, their previous practices in their country of origin have been restricted (Meñaca, 2007b). However, migrants do not put emphasis on these losses. They do not look worried when they talk about them. Traditional technologies/experts take a secondary place both in migrants' parcels and in the professionals contacted in their visits to Ecuador.

This paper is based on the ethnographic data collected during four years of fieldwork in both Spain and Ecuador that formed part of my PhD dissertation (Meñaca, 2007b). In both countries I carried out participant observation in Primary Health care Centres and amongst migrant families. I also interviewed health care professionals (8), migrants (30) and some of their relatives in Ecuador (23). In as many cases as possible, migrants were interviewed repeatedly during these four years. There were three characteristics common to all the migrants in the sample: 1) They travelled to Spain between 2000 and 2003 and had at least one contact waiting for them in Spain. All of them were part of the second big Ecuadorian migration (Jockish and Pribilsky, 2002). 2) All the migrants lived in one of the two largest cities in Spain – Madrid or Barcelona. There was no reference to migration to rural areas. 3) None of the migrants defined him/herself as indigenous.

## A question emerges from the fieldwork data

By the end of the second stage of fieldwork in Ecuador, I was present at the distribution of the parcels sent by a migrant to her family when her brother explained: 'Here, they send us mainly clothes, while (from Ecuador) we send them food and medicines'. It was not the first time I was confronted with the main question that emerged from my fieldwork data: why do migrant families send pharmaceuticals from Ecuador to Spain? In the research design I stated that biomedicine is the hegemonic health model in Ecuador, but I also wrongly assumed that medical technologies were transmitted only in one direction: from Western countries to other parts of the world, and, in this case, from Spain to Ecuador. As fieldwork developed, the evidence became stronger. Medicines were not the only Ecuadorian biomedical resource used by these families. Some migrants used their trips to Ecuador to visit different doctors. From that moment, I began to develop different partial explanations.

The first anthropological explanation was related to the role of parcels and gifts between migrants and their relatives, and thus, a possible social use of medicines in this context. Medicines have a strong symbolic potential, with a clear relation to caring, that can help to strengthen the links within the transnational family. Nevertheless, this power says nothing about the direction of the fluxes. They can be either from the arrival country to the country of origin as in the case of the Soninke migrants in France (Mendiguren, 2006) or from the country of origin to the arrival country, as in my data.

There could be an economic reason. This is what happens with dentists. In Spain dental care is not included in the Public Health System. Ecuadorian migrants take the opportunity to access cheaper dental care in their visits to their country of origin. The strategy is even clearer in families with a long migratory tradition. They know how expensive dentists are in Spain and so, when organising the journey of a new link in the migratory chain, they include a dental revision as part of the preparations. However, the same does not happen with medicines. In Spain pharmaceuticals are cheaper than in Ecuador as they are subsidised by the Public Health care System, but they are mainly sent from Ecuador to Spain.

In the case of medicines, part of the explanation is related to the regulations for their usage. Both in Spain and Ecuador self-medication is a common practice, note that Spain has one of the highest consumption of medicines in Europe (Girona-Brumós *et al.*, 2006). Nevertheless, the control of pharmaceuticals is higher in Spain than in Ecuador, where it is quite easy to obtain medicines, and even those that theoretically need a medical prescription can be bought without it, as observed on several occasions during fieldwork. Migrants also refer to this difference:

> Here (in Spain) they do not sell you remedies directly ... everything must be with a prescription (woman from Guayaquil, 30-40 years old, working class).

> Sometimes I feel tired, but well ... everyday I cook soups and I eat a lot of broccoli, those things help quite a lot ... and the vitamins ... sent by my family, from Ecuador ... I do not buy them here because sometimes, in the drugstores, they do not want to sell us lots of vitamins if not on prescription (woman from Guayaquil, 20-30 years old, middle class).

There are also limits to this argument. Not all the migrants from my sample found it difficult to buy the medicines they needed, and most of the time they did not ask for medicines that required a prescription in Spanish pharmacies, but for painkillers, anti-flu medicines, or vitamins. For another woman, it was a lack of knowledge that made her resort to Ecuadorian medicines 'in the beginning', but later she had no problems buying the medicine she needed:

> In the beginning ... I asked (the family in Ecuador) for aspirins, "characoles" – something we have there, for the flu. In the beginning ... because I didn't know that they could be found here ... Nowadays, I go to the drugstore and ask for something for pain, and they give it to me. In the beginning ... because I didn't know if they would sell us pills in the pharmacy, but now I know, I go and say "it's aching" and they give me something (woman from Quito, 30-40 years old, working class).

In fact, knowledge, familiarity and trust are other possible explanations, but I am not entirely convinced. The migrants that most frequently go to the doctor in Ecuador, or ask their families to send them medicine, are not those who have just arrived in Spain but those who have been there for over five years. As such there is little evidence to support the argument that with greater familiarity and better knowledge of the arrival country's health care system, the demand decreases. On the other hand, those who receive pills from Ecuador and/or attend Ecuadorian doctors during their visits are also using the Spanish health care system. They do utilise Spanish emergency services, hospitals and primary health care centres. One kind of practice does not exclude the other. In general, Ecuadorian migrants use the biomedical resources of both countries.

There are two other important explanations. During fieldwork, migrants based their opinions on the Spanish health care system and justified their transnational practices by focusing on two main points. First of all, they evaluated whether a 'solution' had been given in the terms of biomedical technologies that had cured / 'worked'.[3] Secondly, they referred to the personal interactions with health care professionals that they had experienced. In the following sections I will focus on the first point, I will explain further the migrants' search for technological solutions. I consider this is the key argument for understanding the different practices of migrant families, their multiple uses and evaluations of both Spanish and Ecuadorian biomedical resources.

The analysis must be framed in the plurality within biomedicine. Differences can be found between the biomedical systems of different countries,

as each one has a specific historical development. There are other characteristics that differ depending on whether resource is public or private. Other
distinctions are related to the different biomedical specialisms: in a simple
categorisation, sufficient for the purposes of this paper, I will distinguish
between hospital and primary health care practices.

## In the hospital

In general, migrants' first impression of the Spanish health care system
was positive (Las Heras, 2002). However, their evaluations became more
complex with increasing contact with the health care system. These contacts
were the result of everyday health problems or accidents and emergencies.
It was only then that the distinction between hospital and primary health
centre practices appeared.

Some migrants experienced situations where hospital care was required
and the use of medical technologies was essential to cure, to improve the
quality of life, or to keep people alive – accidents, renal insufficiency, problems of blood coagulation, eye problems, etc. Their discourses about the
attention received from the Spanish health care system in those cases were
centred on the quality of the care and on the fact that it was delivered at
no cost:

> I came here to find out more about my disease, there I was only diabetic.
> (…) My disease affected my heart, lungs, and respiratory truck, all that was
> harmed by swelling. I was examined for endocrine disease, for the heart, for
> the eyes … I have no complaints about the treatment. (…) When they focus
> on my kidneys, they sent me to the hospital. (…) In the beginning, as I am
> not insured, my son, so much money! But they told me not to worry, that
> social insurance would pay, I feel so grateful for that, so grateful. (…) They
> gave me different tests; I admired all the things they have in Bellvitge Hos-
> pital: for the stomach, for the heart, for the kidney (…) I have no complaints
> about the medicine or about the attention I received, in my country I would
> have died. There, dialysis is expensive, it costs $100, and that is what one
> earns, not more. With a public salary, a stable job, one can earn $100 per
> week, not more. If you have to go to dialysis three times per week, it is not
> enough, you die, you die. I admire the social security here, it is widespread,
> for everybody ("Costa" man, over 50 years old, working class).

Geographical inequalities become clear within this category. In Ecuador, when similar situations occur, the cost of medical treatment, which can reach thousands of dollars, is high compared with the average salary of under five hundred dollars per month. Families have to pawn or sell their possessions, such as cars, land or homes. Unfortunately, sometimes this is even not enough and people cannot afford to pay for medical attention, leading to more serious outcomes, even death.

## 'Everyday' health care attention

In the context of 'everyday' medical attention, which is received mainly in health centres, the evaluation of the Spanish health care system was not so positive. Migrants showed discontent with paediatric, gynaecological and adult primary health consultations. The next excerpt is from an interview with the mother of a 5 year old girl who received surgical attention because of a skin problem. She was very happy with the care received in the hospital, but not with the medicine the paediatrician prescribed for flu:

> … (Interviewer: 'and are you happy with the medicine here?')
>
> Yes … well, not with the medicine, but very happy with my daughter's surgery. (…) For the flu or so on, I do not like these medicines here, they do nothing, they have no effect. My daughter has had a serious flu for two months. I was worried. I was going to the paediatrician every week. She was giving me more and more remedies, and nothing helped. I asked my mother in Ecuador, my sister sent me something and it worked. I do not like the medicines here. I think they are to calm, not to heal, not to cure (woman from Quito, 30-40 years old, working class).

Another mother, with a great deal of experience of Spanish emergency and primary health care services, described another situation that ended with a request for medicine, in this case vitamins, from Ecuador:

> My son has suffered lots of things … once they told me he had anaemia, they just told me, they didn't prescribe any vitamin, nothing. I had to make my family send these medicines: vitamins, iron, these things, and look, I have cured him without going to the doctor ("Costa" woman, 20-30 years old, working class).

The complaints included: cases in which no medicine was prescribed to cure a recognised health problem; the small variety of drugs available for children; the small quantity that is usually given; and the inefficacy of the most commonly proposed medicines.

These are the reasons why Ecuadorian migrants consider Spanish common biomedicine less advanced than the Ecuadorian one, where there is a greater variety of medicines available, including those for children, and where medicines are more efficient and completely cure diseases. From their point of view, a doctor must always turn to medical technologies – mainly medicines – to analyse and solve a health problem. Ecuadorian migrants do not expect to be treated by a doctor who does not intervene, who plays down the problem, who explains that it is necessary to wait, that 'in some days' or 'with good nutrition' the problem will disappear.

Similar discontent was encountered relating to primary health attention to adults:

> My health, in the beginning was ok. Later I got sick, the liver, it is killing me. They did an analysis, but the only thing they told me is that it had fat, but they didn't prescribe anything, no painkillers, nothing. I consider they didn't attend very well to me, not at all. The GP didn't do a proper revision, he gave a report, and nothing else, to the specialist. And the specialist… what they told me was that my liver had fat and that it had grown. But nothing, nothing, nothing. Just not to eat fat or acidic foods. (…) I have other problems with menstruation, and they tell me they don't know what I have, and it's not possible, not having anything but menstruation is not coming. They have told me they will phone me to do another analysis, but until now they haven't. I think I will visit a doctor in Ecuador. It might be the climate, or nerves, or stress. I want to get attended to there. Here, they don't say what it is that I have (woman from Quito, 20-30 years old, working class).

An important part of the negative vision offered by the Ecuadorian migrants is related to the 'lack of solution'. The 'lack of solution' when they do not receive more than advice about nutrition and hygiene, when they are not given medicines, when the prescriptions are always the same inefficient ones, or when doctors say that 'intervening or not intervening will have the same result'. In the worst cases, they are not even given a diagnosis, doctors say they 'do not see anything', and/or not enough clinical tests are carried out to understand, in depth, the causes of the problem.

There is a difference in the attention given to adults compared with that given to children. Whilst most of children's problems are presented to doctors as obvious symptoms – fever, cough, runny nose – and there is no doubt about the biological origins of the problem, this is not the case for the physical complaints of adults. Most of the examples that were described during fieldwork referred to problems for which biomedicine is not able to find a specific biological cause: cronified cystitis, dermatological complaints, unspecific pains in different parts of the body – liver, heart, ovaries – or the whole body, 'I am feeling so bad', and even a case of fybromialgia. The interpretation of different health professionals includes a possible 'psychosomatic' origin: the physical disorder could be the result of the somatisation of the different social problems, worries, stress, and/ or anguish the migrants might suffer. It is not that migrants are the only group of patients that present psychosomatic complaints (García-Campayo *et al.*, 1996; Lobo *et al.*, 1996): generally, primary health care practitioners consider that their users do not bring pertinent problems to the consultation when they come 'on demand' (Uribe, 1996). Nevertheless, particular attention has been given to immigrants' health complaints, and it has been argued that they are more prone to somatisation than North Europeans or North Americans, due to their different health seeking processes and their idioms of distress (van Moffaert and Vereecken, 1989; Bäärnhielm and Ekbald, 2000; van Dijk and van Dongen, 2000).

I do not want to reflect on the social origin of migrants' distress, but to point out when the psychosomatic model is integrated into the biomedical discourse: biomedicine employs psychosomatic explanations, describing how the mind could affect the body and produce distress, mainly in those cases where no physical cause is detected (Cohn, 1999; Tosal, 2003). This process generates conflict and disagreement between doctors and, in this case, the migrant patients: neither group considers the others actions appropriate. Health professionals find the worries and demands of users of tests or medicines unjustified, while patients find the responses given by the doctor inappropriate. They attend consultations for a diagnosis, an in-depth analysis, a treatment and a cure, that they do not receive. Users on the one hand continue with the logic of biologic reductionism and technological progress that defines biomedicine, while doctors, on the other hand, not being able to give a response from their 'own' logic, resort to psychosomatic explanations, discrediting patients' demands and experiences.

In their search for other health care alternatives, Ecuadorian migrants continue to follow the hegemonic biomedical logic. They resort to Ecuadorian medicines. Vitamins, antibiotics, anti-flu, orthopaedic shoes, anti-parasite drugs, eczema lotions, etc. are sent to them by their relatives, still resident in Ecuador, on demand. They consult Ecuadorian doctors during their holidays. Their visits to private specialists can become one of the main objectives of, and activities during, their trips to Ecuador.

Most of the time, but not always, the solution to the health problem is sought in Ecuador. Spanish private medicine is also considered an option, though often unaffordable for most migrant families. Migrants that send about 200€ to their families in Ecuador each month – an amount that significantly improves the quality of life in their country of origin – will not spend over 60€ for just one medical consultation.

## Conclusion: Ecuadorian migrants' embodiment of the hegemonic biomedical model

In the context of migration, Ecuadorian migrant families increasingly access different biomedical services. This variability in the use of biomedical resources does not make reference to multiple health care logics, but just to the central biomedical one. The biological reductionism and the self-image of scientific and technological progress are two central characteristics of the biomedical self-definition (Kleinman, 1995; Menéndez, 2005). Ecuadorian migrants have embodied this model and value the specificity of biomedicine. They expect biomedical professionals to cure their health problems using efficient technologies, both in hospitals and in primary health care centres.

In general, in hospital interventions they find what they were looking for: advanced technologies for diagnosis and cure. The limitations to the success of biomedicine are, in this case, enforced by a lack of access. In Ecuador there are situations when the required health care facilities are not available in more economical and/or public hospitals, whilst they are not affordable in the private hospitals that offer them. Amongst the primary health care providers, the Spanish public health centres are the main places where the expected response is not found (Table 1.)

| | Hospital | | Primary Health | |
|---|---|---|---|---|
| | Public | Private | Public | Private |
| Ecuador | – | ++<br>but not affordable | + | ++ |
| Spain | ++ | no data | – – | + |

**Table 1.** *Ecuadorian migrants' technological evaluation of the different biomedical services*

Public sector primary health care practitioners in Spain would not consider the provision of more antibiotics, vitamins, anti-parasite drugs, orthopaedic shoes, or the carrying out of unnecessary diagnostic tests as more technological and efficient. They consider that it has been scientifically demonstrated that it is not useful and can even be iatrogenic. The debate is complex, therefore we should put in perspective both migrants' voices and doctors' scientific truth.

Doctors are not listening to the migrants who clearly state that they find no total cure in the doctors advice and medicines. They are ignoring the fact that healing is not limited to biology, and that medicines have more than a biological effect. Doctors are not taking into consideration the variability within their colleagues' prescriptions. This variability does not only appear between public and private practitioners, but also between professionals working within the same sector. Protocols are not unique or unambiguous, and doctors' interpretations and agreement with them depends largely on their clinical experiences. Last but not least, doctors 'forget' that these new practices of reducing prescriptions in the public health care sector are closely associated with the efforts and pressure from the health authorities to reduce health costs, and in particular pharmaceutical costs; common strategies which developed in the context of the economic and welfare state crisis of the eighties.

On the other hand, we could say that Ecuadorian migrants are 'technologically fascinated' (Peiró and Bernal-Delgado, 2006). They are not the only ones. Industry, medical professionals and patients interact and are all responsible for the growing intensity in the use of technologies, independently of their value or their iatrogenic effects (Puig-Junoy, 2006; Gervás, 2006). From this critical perspective, it could be said that Ecuadorian migrants' discourses and practices are mainly a new example of the narrow space left by the hegemonic model for other (new?) health models that do not have such a biological and technological core, such as Alma Ata's primary health care proposals.

In these pages I have shown how the unexpected health practices of migrant families – the resort to Ecuadorian medicines and health professionals – are more related to a shared central logic than to a multiplicity of medical realities. However, it has also been shown how a central organising principle can lead to a diversity of health practices depending on previous experiences, the fluid web of resources and the social relations one cultural group shares. The specificity of the Ecuadorian migrants' pragmatics of health care must also be acknowledged. In a context were migration is being 'medicalised' – considered the cause of different mental health problems – and migrants' body complaints are regarded as 'psychosomatic', migrants' practices of relaying in Ecuadorian biomedicine allow them first of all to find 'a cure', an answer to their complaints, but also, to continue and strengthen relations with the country of origin; to re-evaluate their country of origin as one with more technological and modern biomedical resources, and to confront Spanish GP suggestions that tend towards the 'psychiatrisation' of their condition. Migrants do have an active role taking care of their health. An active practice by which they 'resist' the different attempts found both in the country of origin and arrival (Meñaca, 2008), i.e. to 'medicalise'/'psychiatrise' migration.

## Notes

1   This paper is based on my PhD dissertation. I am grateful to the Spanish Ministry of Education for the FPU scholarship, which supported my work in association with the EU financed projects 'Partners for Health, I and II'. In Ecuador, I received much support from both FLACSO University and CEAS. I would also like to thank my PhD supervisors – Rosario Otegui, Josep M. Comelles and Els van Dongen – for their advice during the whole process; the members of my PhD tribunal, the participants in the MAAH conference, and the peer reviewers of this text for their relevant input; and Natalie Evans and Christopher Pell for supervising and correcting my English.

2   Subaltern medicines are not compact, nor independent, nor homogeneous realities, on the contrary: they combine and distribute themselves in a complex mosaic (Bartoli, 2005). Using the categories that my informants have distinguished, they include practices held not only by professionals or people with a specific knowledge, but also by the families. The most common categories are traditional nosologies –mainly *susto* and *ojeadura*- and homemade remedies, most of my informants talked about them. Other alternative medicines used by the families in Ecuador include professionals

and shops that use/sell different herbs or remedies made by herbs in a mixture of tradition and cosmopolitism, Chinese medicine, and sorcerers. Although there is international acknowledgment of the *otavalo / quichwa* medicine (Knipper, 2006), none of my informants gave me references of consultation with a *yachak / chamán*, which could be related to the fact that none of them defined him or herself as an indigenous.

3    In this chapter, it is not my intention to analyse the mechanisms involved in this perceived efficacy. The anthropology of pharmaceuticals (van der Geest, Reynolds Whyte and Hardon, 1996; Reynolds Whyte, van der Geest and Hardon, 2002) provides an excellent framework to understand the social and symbolic mechanisms involved in the efficacy of the medicines. However, in this specific case that kind of analysis remains to be done.

## Bibliography

Bäärnhielm, S. and S. Ekblad (2000). Turkish migrant women encountering health care in Stockholm: a qualitative study of somatization and illness meaning. *Culture, Medicine and Psychiatry* 24: 431-452.

Bartoli, P. (2005). ¿Esperando al doctor? Reflexiones sobre una investigación de antropología médica en México. *Revista de Antropología Social* 14: 71-100.

Burke, N. (2007). Book review. *American Anthropologist* 109 (3): 545-546.

Carvalho, C. (2006). Exporting therapies: how Guinean therapists are making their way in a globalised market. *9th EASA Biennial Conference 'Europe and the World'*. Bristol: EASA.

Cohn, S. (1999). Taking time to smell the roses: accounts of people with Chronic Fatigue Syndrome and their struggle for legitimisation. *Anthropology and Medicine* 6 (2): 195-215.

Comelles, J.M. (2004). El regreso de las culturas. Diversidad y práctica médica en el s. XXI. En Fernández Juárez, G. (coord.) *Salud e interculturalidad en América Latina*, pp. 17-30. Quito: Ediciones Abya-Yala – Agencia BOLHISPANA – Universidad de Castilla-La Mancha.

García-Campayo, J., R. Campos, G. Marcos, M.J. Pérez-Echevarría, A. Lobo and GMPPZ (1996). Somatisation in primary care in Spain II. Differences between somatisers and psychologisers. *British Journal of Psychiatry* 168: 348-353.

Gervás, J. (2006). Moderación en la actividad médica preventiva y curativa. Cuatro ejemplos de necesidad de prevención cuaternaria en España. *Gaceta Sanitaria* 20 (Supl. 1): 127-134.

Girona-Brumós, L., R. Ribera-Montañá, J.C. Juárez-Giménez and M.P. Lalueza-Broto (2006). Luces y sombras de la prestación farmacéutica en España: a propósito de los antidepresivos y antipsicóticos. *Gaceta Sanitaria* 20 (Supl. 1): 143-153.

González, B., R.M. Urbanos and P. Ortega (2004). Oferta pública y privada de servicios sanitarios por comunidades autónomas. *Gaceta Sanitaria* 18 (Supl. 1): 82-89.

Hahn, R. and A. Kleinman (1983). Biomedical practical and anthropological theory: frameworks and directions. *Annual Review of Anthropology* 12: 305-333.

Jokisch, B.D. and J. Pribilsky (2002). The panic to leave: economic crisis and the 'new' emigration from Ecuador. *International Migration* 40 (4): 75-101.

Kangas, B. (2002). Therapeutic itineraries in a global world: Yemenis and their search for biomedical treatment abroad. *Medical Anthropology* 21(1): 35-78.

Kim, M.Y., H.R. Han, K.B. Kim and D.N. Duong (2002). The use of traditional and western medicine among Korean American elderly. *Journal of Community Health* 27 (2): 109-120.

Kleinman, A. (1995). *Writing at the margin. Discourse between Anthropology and Medicine.* Berkeley: University of California Press.

Knipper, M. (2006). El reto de la 'medicina intercultural' y la historia de la 'medicina tradicional' indígena contemporánea. G. Fernández Juárez (coord.) *Salud e interculturalidad en America Latina. Antropología de la salud y crítica intercultural.* Quito – Toledo: Abya Yala – Universidad de Castilla-La Mancha.

Las Heras Mosteiro, J. (2002). *El proceso asistencial y la utilización de los servicios sanitarios por la población inmigrante irregular. El discurso del colectivo ecuatoriano.* PhD Thesis. Madrid: Facultad de Medicina, Universidad Autónoma de Madrid.

LaVeist, Thomas A. (2005). *Minority populations and health. An introduction to health disparities in the United States.* San Francisco: Jossey-Bass.

Lobo, A., J. García-Campayo, R. Campos, G. Marcos, M.J. Pérez-Echevarría and GMPPZ (1996). Somatisation in primary care in Spain. Estimates of prevalence and clinical characteristics. *British Journal of Psychiatry*, 168: 344-348.

Ma, G.X. (1999). Between two worlds: The use of traditional and Western health services by Chinese immigrants. *Journal of Community Health* 24 (6): 421-437.

Mendiguren, B. (2006). *Inmigración, medicalización y cambio social entre los Soninke: el caso de Dramané (Mali, África).* PhD Thesis. Tarragona: DAFITS, Universitat Rovira i Virgili.

Menéndez, E. (2005).Intencionalidad, experiencia y función: la articulación de los saberes médicos. *Revista de Antropología Social* 14: 33-69.

Meñaca, A. (2006). Familias rotas y problemas de salud. La medicalización de las familias migrantes ecuatorianas. *Quaderns 22:161-178.* Barcelona, ICA.

Meñaca, A. (2007a). Sistema Sanitario e inmigración. El papel de la cultura. In: M.L. Esteban (ed.), *Introducción a la Antropología de la Salud. Aplicaciones teóricas y prácticas.* Bilbo: OSALDE – OP.

Meñaca, A. (2007b). *Antropología, salud y migraciones. Procesos de autocuidado en familias migrantes ecuatorianas.* PhD Thesis. Tarragona: Departament d'Antropolgia, Filosofia i Treball Social. Facultat de Lletres. Universitat Rovira i Virgili.

O.P.S. (2001). *Perfil del sistema de servicios de salud de Ecuador.* Programa de Organización y Gestión de Sistemas y Servicios de Salud, División de Desarrollo de Sistemas y Servicios de Salud, Organización Panamericana de la Salud.

Peiró, S. and E. Bernal-Delgado (2006). ¿A qué incentivos responde la utilización hospitalaria en el Sistema Nacional de Salud? *Gaceta Sanitaria* 20 (Supl. 1): 110-116.

Puig-Junoy, J. (2006). ¿Es la financiación sanitaria suficiente y adecuada? *Gaceta Sanitaria* 20 (Supl. 1): 96-102.

Reynolds Whyte, S., S. van der Geest and A. Hardon (2002). *Social lives of medicines.* Cambridge: Cambridge University Press.

Tiilikainen, M. (2006). Transnational healing practices: Some considerations based on fieldwork in Northern Somalia. *4th Biennial Conference of the European Network of Medical Anthropology at Home*. Conference paper. Seili: Finlandia.

Tosal, B. (2003). *Histéricas, quejicas y simuladores. El problema de legitimación de la fibromialgia*. Master's Thesis. Tarragona: Universitat Rovira i Virgili, Departament d'Antropologia, Filosofia i Treball Social.

Uribe Oyarbide, J.M. (1996). *Educar y cuidar. El diálogo cultural en atención primaria*. Madrid: Ministerio de Cultura.

van der Geest, S., S. Reynolds Whyte and A. Hardon (1996). The anthropology of pharmaceuticals: a biographical approach. *Annual Review of Anthropology* 25: 153-178.

van Dijk, R. and E. van Dongen (2000). Migrants and health care in the Netherlands. In: P. Vulpiani, J.M. Comelles and E. van Dongen (eds.). *Health for all, all in Health. European experiences on health care for migrants*. Perugia: Cidis/Alisei.

van Dongen, E. (2008). Cancer and integrity. Dealing with fragile realities. *Medical Anthropology at Home 2008*. Conference paper. Sandbjerg: Aarhus University.

van Moffaert, M. and A. Vereecken (1989). Somatization of psychiatric illness in Mediterranean migrants in Belgium. *Culture, Medicine and Psychiatry* 13: 297-213.

Mabel Gracia Arnaiz

Chapter XI.

# Obesity as a Social Problem: Thoughts about its Chronic, Pandemic and Multi-factorial Character

This article shows how the biomedical understanding of obesity and the preventative proposals which have been devised by Spanish institutions during recent decades have helped turn food and body weight into a social problem. Expert constructs regarding obese people, diet and weight control offer valuable information regarding the biomedical understanding of the illness and of current lifestyles, that is, what the nature of these lifestyles is or should be. This text falls within the framework of wider studies which have as their objective to analyse how and why specific eating behaviours have become social problems and the ways in which dietetic norms are constructed.[1] My objective is to reflect briefly on why many of the pragmatic and symbolic reasons which inform the choice and consumption of food have been substituted by other nutritional reasons. Taking obesity as an example, this article will then reflect generally on the medicalisation of contemporary food and weight.

With this aim in mind, I will link Mennell's and Turner's proposals regarding the civilising of the appetite with the relation between the expansion of capitalism and the prescribed managing of the diet and body. I propose to illustrate this by using what I define here as the processes of *dietary and bodily normalisation*, that is the construction, on the one hand, of a specific dietary pattern – the balanced diet – and on the other, of a weight pattern based on the BMI which, by measuring other indicators, establishes what is or is not a normal bodily volume. Both processes share the idea that to promote health, subjects must eat and weigh less, thus creating rules regarding food intake, bodily weight and physical activity. I will try to show, through the problematisation of obesity as an individual responsibility, some of the limitations of interpreting food behaviour principally through the prism of health and illness without taking into account the complex nature of food and culture.

## The construction of *dietary normality*

Eating, a basic biological necessity, becomes a complex process to which humans through social relations give multiple functions and meanings. There are so many varied eating behaviours and they demonstrate and express what it means to eat, what food means to people and why we eat. Eating behaviour, as with other potentially communicative phenomena can be used for ends distinct from procuring subsistence: through the foods we access, accept or reject we can manifest gender and class identities, social inequalities or forms of resistance to adverse situations. It is like this in all cultures, and ours is no exception. We can demonstrate gratitude, acceptance, interest or status in respect to guests, family or friends, distributing food or sharing meals with them. For this we eat certain foods, often different and more abundant on special occasions such as religious festivals, personal events and local celebrations (Powdermarker, 1997). The abundant Roman banquets and the practice of vomiting reflected the excesses that the rich aristocracy were permitted, just as in the Middle Ages English nobles and landowners sat at their tables and had feasts consisting of twenty or thirty different dishes of meat of diverse types with the socio-political purpose of symbolising the power they exercised over plain folks (Fieldhouse, 1996: 79-80). Generosity expressed through food is still today important in numerous societies. On islands in the Pacific, food is prepared in great quantities with the expectation that one or more guests may turn up: 'A good meal is that in which, upon finishing, all the participants remark that they are very full and have enjoyed excellent company' (Pollock, 2000:46).

These habits show that eating practices are not only governed by biological necessity to fill the body with fuel, which is a mechanistic vision of the human organism (Vigarello, 2006), but rather by the material conditions and the symbolic representations expressed in social relations in different societies. Consequently, it is worth questioning the logic which underlies copious or restrictive food consumption and relate this to how in Western societies eating a lot, a little or nothing is readily attributed to the anomalous or pathological character of an individual.

Taking these examples into account, it might be surprising that nowadays modern discussion about food behaviours by political authorities and health experts is couched above all in terms of health and illness, and that food behaviours have become a medical responsibility. Really, however, this should come as no surprise. Western medicine has a long tradition of providing information and advice regarding the quantity and composition of healthy food, the regulation of weight and the prevention of illnesses and this has helped the biological function of foods to become predominant over the course of time. Also, thanks to the influence of Western medicine, the biological function of food is predominant in other medical systems as well.

The fact that a biomedical interpretation emphasises the physiological at the expense of the social is the result of a way of thinking whose development has gone hand in hand with the medicalisation food (Sobal, 1995). This latter process has its origins in classical Antiquity in Hippocratic treatises which popularised the maxim *let your food be your medicine*, and in Galenic medicine, and in the medieval *regimina sanitatis*, when speaking about how people should care for their bodies and health (Manzini, 1996; Barona 2008). Later on, dietary rules were applied to try to get people to choose and consume food more for medical rather than for pragmatic or symbolic reasons (Poulain, 2002). The influence of mechanistic theory meant this tendency became more accentuated in the 17th and 18th centuries and that more attention was paid to the healthy qualities of foods. The well-known English physicist, George Cheyne (1733) referred to the body (an instrument made up of circuits and fluxes) using a mechanical metaphor which described food as the fuel which supplied the human machine. He also stated that a rich diet, such as the sumptuous diet of the elite, was the origin of numerous illness and should, therefore, be modified.

The 19th century saw food being produced in larger quantities and distributed more evenly in Western countries, and this coincided with successive food reforms designed to limit excessive food consumption (Levenstein, 1996). It was during this period that what Mennell (1985), following Elías (1989), called the civilising of appetite became very evident. According to Mennell, this process took place over several centuries and was the means by which behavioural norms were modified in a specific way. That is, the gradual civilising of the appetite was a progressive change from the individual being subject to principally external constraints (which may be, for example, ecological, economic or symbolic) towards the individual developing and exercising internal constraints (such as diet, hygiene).

Thus, for example, in Christian areas, and specifically Protestant ones, dietary recommendations came to form part of an ethical standpoint. According to these recommendations, caring for the body was a moral responsibility which established, as Turner (1982, 1999) puts it, a parallel between the optional management of the diet and the expansion of capitalism. Dietary restrictions prevented gluttony among the elite, whereas a sufficiently nutritious diet maintained the workers and therefore the workforce. In the

U.S.A. these principals were preached in the homes of the working classes by representatives of *New Nutrition*, a group of nutritionists, social reformers and specialists in home economics who wanted to organise the workers' food expenditure by changing, without much success, their cooking habits (Levenstein, 1996).

According to Barona (2008: 87-88), nutrition became a common element of culture, economy and health when the state emerged as a social regulator and food production and consumption became a state responsibility. In the twentieth century nutrition expertise and scientific knowledge became a major concern for most European governments, for civil society and for social and charitable organisations as a consequence of international conflicts and market crises. Hunger and poverty were considered social and public health problems and the provision of food became a basic human right, endowed with a moral dimension: dietary habits and traditional agricultural production schemes could have negative effects on both health and economy and on the common good and had to be modified. The idea of an optimum diet based on physiological research on calorie intake and expenditure and on protein, fat, mineral and vitamin requirements was introduced at that time. This signified the origin of the standardisation of methods used in dietary studies as well as the standardisation of food patterns between countries and rural and urban populations: 'the role of nutritional experts not only influences knowledge, but also inspires agriculture and health policies, education and propaganda programmes, aimed at disciplining and changing popular habits' (Barona 2008: 88). Thus, during the 20th century health and nutrition had become essential factors for the making of citizenship, implying changing relationships between state, society and individuals.

Currently, *dietary normalisation* is centred on the balanced diet, that is, it is a feeding pattern based on restricting or promoting the consumption of certain foods[2] – what and how much to eat – and on prescribing a set of guidelines related to how, when with whom to do this. The aim of this is a healthy nutrition 'free from health risks'.[3] Nevertheless, these objectives involve normalising daily life (Conveney, 2006). Indeed, this is the aim of the various guides published to promote a healthy diet (Dapcich et al. 2004, Aranceta 2002, Generalitat de Catalunya 2005) when they try to teach the individual how to eat well. That is, when they advise the individual to eat in the company of others, not to eat too slowly nor too fast, to chew slowly, to eat between three and five times a day at well defined times, to eat a variety of foods in the right quantities, they are promoting a way of regulating lifestyles which is based on a responsibility to care for oneself and which demands true dietary competence (Ascher, 2005). I will now look at these questions in terms of the medicalisation of food and corpulence in Western societies.

## Obesity as a multifactorial, pandemic and chronic illness

The progressive, although not recent, process by which the issue of weight has been turned into a social problem (Poulain, 2000) has involved cultural criteria such as regarding gluttony with contempt or venerating thinness and, more recently, has involved economic and health criteria such as the negative impact of excess weight on health and healthcare costs.[4] Defined medically as an excessive or abnormal accumulation of fat (Basdevant and Guy-Gran, 2004), obesity is considered today to be a multifactorial and chronic illness which, because of its increasing prevalence worldwide, has reached epidemic proportions (WHO, 2004). However, it can also be prevented by having a 'healthy lifestyle' which maintains a 'balance between calories ingested and calories spent'.[5] Dietary problems, and in particular those related to weight,[6] have often been thought to be caused by the quantity of food ingested, as if the effects on the body of eating were simply a question of arithmetic; that is, if we eat too much or too little we put on or lose weight according to the calories we consume and spend. The reality is less simple, since weight is far from exclusively dependent on the quantities of food ingested. It also depends on hormonal and neural mechanisms and constitutional, metabolic and genetic factors (Alemany, 2003).

Ever since obesity has been associated with increased morbidity and mortality due to non-transmisable chronic illnesses such as hypertension, diabetes or heart attack, and ever since the Body Mass Index (BMI)[7] has become established, not without controversy (Sobal and Stunkard 1990; Basdevant and Guy-Gran, 2004), as the most widely used indicator for identifying obesity, the whole population has been taught – despite their biosocial heterogeneity – to try and stay within the limits of their BMI by closely watching their weight, having a balanced diet and exercising regularly. In general, this means 'eating less' (Nestlé, 2002) and 'moving more' because nowadays being fat has become, especially in industrialised countries, synonymous with being ill.

According to this medicalised view of excess weight and obesity, it is taken as self evident (although it is not in reality) that fat kills, that obesity is in itself a pathology, and that all obese people must be ill or will be in the future (Campos, 2004). Obesity is a sign of transgressing the rules and the result of doing something which ought not to be done; that is, eating too much and being idle. The negative perception among health professionals of excess weight often rests on the idea that, once it is established, it is an untreatable illness because of the tendency to continue to put on weight and because of the obese person's supposed lack of interest or willpower in trying to lose weight by dieting or exercising (Maddox and Liederman, 1969).

Although in the field of healthcare there are nutritionists who try to treat the patient as a whole by adapting their advice to the patient's bio, psycho and social particularities (De Labarre, 2004), patients are frequently reproached on moral grounds for their dietary behaviour, and this makes them feel they are irresponsible and lacking in judgement or ability: 'Often…when we don't feel well we compensate for it by eating and drinking, even if we have no appetite and it goes against our better judgement and our health'.[8]

When prescribing diets for losing weight, many doctors believe that their patients are responsible for their own dysfunction (Crawford, 1997; Ryan, 1977): 'If you are obese it is because you *don't know how* or *don't want* to eat well'. In cases where the overweight patients are children, this responsibility is easily transferred to the parents, as has happened recently in Great Britain, where the mother of Connor McCreaddie, a nine year old boy weighing 89 kilos, was on the point of losing custody of her child and was accused of negligence, or in the case of the boy from Asturias (Northern Spain) who, for the same reason, has been separated from his family since June 2006. After being taken into care by the Asturian social services he has lost 40 of his 100 kilos and will not be returned home until 'the family environment encourages the youngster to adopt healthy habits'.[9] Unfortunately, this conception towards fatness being an illness is not only contributing to increase physical and moral panic against excess weight, but is stigmatising obese people even more. It is not surprising that in this context activist and scientific groups have emerged claiming the acceptance of fatness (Saguy y Riley 2005).[10]

Choosing to regard lifestyles as untidy or inadequate because they are the product of a plentiful and decadent civilisation (Gard and Wright, 2006), has not only helped health experts to legitimise their civilising of the appetite, but also to continue the process through the practice of prevention. The argument in favour of nutritional education in the case of obesity is threefold (Ascher 2006): 1) individuals live better if they follow a healthy diet; 2) they work better if they enjoy good health; and 3) they cost less to general society. The moral, economic and health aims of such proposals, therefore, are clear.

However, numerous questions need to be answered about these approaches and, although it is beyond the scope of this article to try to formulate and answer these questions, I will point out some of those which, I think, are the most important. In the first place, is it true that, as is maintained by public health campaigns, consumers do not know how to eat or, to put it another way, do we have bad eating habits? Is it true that dietary behaviours are more unstructured than in previous eras and that this lack of structure affects everybody equally?

Various studies show that the lack of structure regarding eating habits in modern society is only relative, given that even if there has been a simplification and individualisation regarding meals, as well as a slight increase in the number of daily intakes, it is not possible to establish a relationship between these trends and the worsening in people's health (Poulain, 2002; Contreras and Gracia, 2004). To accept the premise that there is a lack of structure regarding eating and that this has negative effects on the population may be useful for legitimising the steps taken in nutritional education, but it does not seem scientifically sustainable. If alimentary and social order really has become degraded, then it is surprising that people's life expectancies have increased dramatically and that this has been attributed, in part, to improved nutrition among certain social groups. For its part, the epidemiological literature shows that eating problems, among them obesity, do not affect everybody equally. Not everybody eats badly and not everybody is fat. In most countries, obesity is most prevalent among the poor. However, few would dare to maintain that the poor eat badly or worse because of a lack of knowledge and skills regarding eating, instead they prefer to refer how difficult it is to gain access to (healthy) food.

Despite the acceptance of explanatory structural factors, weight increase has been associated with the adaptation of individual eating behaviours without taking into account that this nutritional adaptation has varied at different times and in different places. In effect, numerous nutritional recommendations have changed dietary behaviour in favour of improving collective health and have questioned, with greater or lesser wisdom, how beneficial previous habits were, proposing new ones in their place. This was the case, for example, with the contradictory medical prescriptions given throughout the last century in Spain regarding breastfeeding, which arbitrarily undermined maternal abilities (Barona, 2002).

It is well known that what has been considered good or bad, or normal or pathological in terms of health changes through time has varied, and for this reason it is a wise to be prudent when establishing dogmas based on scientific grounds (Tannahill, 1988). In the current highly medicalised context, more and more dietary practices are considered risky or bad because they have been objectified and quantified as such by learned experts (Gracia, 2004). Risk is a concept in modern societies which coincides with statistical calculation and appears when it is thought something can and should be done to avoid a perceived psychic or physical threat.

To believe that avoiding risky behaviours depends, to a large extent, on the individual is to misunderstand, as is argued by Douglas and Wildasky (1983) and Boltanski and Thévenot (1991), that subjects perceive or represent an object or activity as risky depending on their economic or political surroundings, their systems of values and beliefs, and the position they occupy, for reasons of gender, class, age or ethnic group, in a given society. And it is these structural determinants, organised in complex systems, which affect people and which determine for them ultimately whether or not a behaviour is preferable compared with others. Dietary habits are not determined exclusively by our preoccupation with health or illness. There are individuals for whom the risks of putting on weight are not about becoming morbidly obese, but rather about no longer having a socially acceptable body (Lupton, 2000). On the other hand, there are fat people who are not worried by their weight and instead use it as a reason to demand institutional recognition of their particular state (Menéndez, 2002).

## Eating well, eating badly: a reductionist conception of culture and food

Given the diverse meanings attributed to obesity, its different causes and the ways it affects the health of the population, it does not seem sensible to consider it to be the result of irresponsibly adopting risky behaviours.[11] In general terms, it is thought that excess weight and obesity have directly resulted from changes in social habits in general and from the worsening of diets in particular. All this leads Western nutritional experts to emphasise, again, the importance of the relationship between diet and health. It has also led to the proliferation of guides and standards for eating well and to recurring warnings to the public about the need to have a sensible diet, to eat less and to do more exercise in order to stay healthy.

In Spain, the current model applies the principal that in order to modify bad habits and eliminate the non-rational reasons which guide dietary preferences, it is both necessary and a priority to improve the public's dietary knowledge. This is explicitly set out in the health authorities' strategy for dealing with obesity: 'The family, as the principle transmitter of messages, should have a basic knowledge of what constitutes a healthy diet which in turn allows them to create varied and balanced meals'.[12] All the dietary guides point in the same direction. If it is accepted that '[dietary] habits begin around three or four years of age, are established by the age of eleven and consolidated throughout the individual's life',[13] the act of exercising control over food is legitimised at a younger and younger age and begins with the first meal of the day, breakfast: 'it is necessary to spend between 15 and 20 minutes on breakfast, sitting at the table, with the family if possible, in a relaxed environment ...'[14]

In this strategy, obesity is defined as an evil arising from the individual's immediate environment which must be approached 'without resorting to a repressive campaign, interpreted by the citizen as prescriptive or prohibitive',[15] whilst also understanding that 'a person's surroundings play a primordial role in the development of the global obesity epidemic by creating the so-called obesogenic environment'.[16] Collective initiatives have been put forward, on paper at least, proposing the participation of the various social agents involved, such as schools, the food industry, public administrations or health professionals.

However, we must ask ourselves why the steps promoted by prevention programmes have had a minimal effect on the socioeconomic environment, whilst other steps directed at the individual continue to be promoted. The methods for attaining so-called healthy lifestyles continue to be centred on modifying personal behaviour, such as, for example, reaching an energy balance and a normal weight, improving nutritional knowledge or increasing physical activity. Efforts have been made in these fields for some time now but success has been somewhat modest (Farré, 2005).

This is because, in our opinion, the steps proposed have not taken into account the complex nature of either eating behaviour or culture. Why do they urge people to modify their inappropriate dietary habits whilst not proposing effective measures for changing a system which, when all is said and done, encourages the emergence of certain illnesses in certain social groups? Furthermore, nutritional recommendations should not forget that epidemilogical studies show that in many countries obesity is higher in women than in men and higher among poor and less well educated people (Sobal, 2001; Aranceta et al. 2005; Barquera, 2006). Therefore, why continue to send out standardised messages about the suitability of the balanced diet as it is currently understood if, for cultural or structural reasons, many people cannot gain access to it?

On the other hand, when looking for the causes or agents of particular problems, the social environment should not be defined, as is the case with many institutions, as some kind of nebulous abstract (obesogenic environment or favourable environment) making it, therefore, difficult to approach, but rather it should be understood as a product of society itself (Gracia and Contreras, 2008).

In industrialised societies, this means understanding the political, economic and cultural determinants which are associated with consumer capitalism. There is a need to reconsider the use of culture in the diagnosis relating to the deterioration of our eating habits. Fast food, passive leisure, central heating, motorised transport, deficiency of sports facilities, food advertisements…have, amongst many others, been established as the causal agents. It is relatively easy to enumerate possible social-cultural reasons in the origin and evolution of obesity, but it is more difficult to prove them. All of these factors are present in our societies, but there is hardly any knowledge as to whether these influence daily life, or if this influence has been negative.

In the light of this we may ask: To combat obesity why not reduce the prices of healthy food, dispose of junk food and improve the opportunities for the poor? Isn't it unhealthy to work long days, be paid a low salary and carry out a variety of incompatible activities? We have little knowledge on the effects of these factors. We know, however, that the actual strategies have not been designated to incorporate these or other social needs. On the contrary, a good part of prevention campaigns are structured on the basic concept of culture and eating habits: it is possible to change them by adopting correct dietetic behaviours. The social and cultural factors are understood to be the specific agents that cause illness or death and which can be treated individually.

Lang and Rayner (2007) suggest that the moment has arrived to re-think public health. Therefore to avoid a political cacophony derived from different explanatory models of obesity, they propose an alternative approach that has less effect on matters such as, eat more or eat less, modify food labels or give nutritional information – and greater effect with regard to the more difficult issues of linking the physical, physiological, social and cognitive fields in different ways and degrees, within the basic health and illness process.

## Conclusion

Although obesity is presented as an indisputable global problem, the social and anthropological literature stresses the need to recognise its condition of social construct, and to contextualise its origin in dynamic processes. In the explanatory models of obesity, there are not many interdisciplinary approaches that contribute to the better understanding of its nature and dimensions. There are reflective proposals missing that incorporate the historicity of the processes that conform and articulate the different levels involved.

Expert constructs about diet and excess of weight do not merely offer valuable information about the nature and possible effects of some medical practices designed to try and change the disorganised lifestyles which progress and civilisation have brought us. They also offer information about how these constructs help to produce and maintain patterns for promoting health which, despite the economic and cultural diversity of different populations, are very similar at a global level. One of the paradoxes about the medicalisation of diet in industrialised societies is that, on the one hand, the idea of the balanced diet has penetrated the social network and has even given some basis to irreverent discussions about what it is to eat well, while, on the other hand, its accompanying food practices have not managed to catch on. This is demonstrated by the increase in chronic illnesses linked to obesity.

What is surprising about the occurrence of obesity is that it has increased despite the fact that aesthetic models encourage contempt for excess weight; despite efforts by the health authorities to teach healthy habits; and, despite the food industry not reducing its efforts to offer products, many of them for controlling weight. However, the explanation can be found, at least in part, in the construction of contexts which discursively are so inopportune, but which in practice are so encouraging. There are many studies which warn of the consequences of repeated medical recommendations and the commercial and social pressures to avoid excess weight and obesity which have caused people from the earliest times to go on diets and enter a vicious circle of weight loss and weight gain. They also warn of the consequences of a society whose transformed structure now demands more and more sedentary occupations which are also more and more diversified, where following the routine laid down by good dietary advice becomes very difficult.

This divergence between normative knowledge and dietary practices brings into question, to a large extent, the efficacy of the current model of nutritional prevention and intervention, principally for two reasons. The first reason is that little work is being done on structural factors which might explain the increase in the prevalence of obesity, such as, for example, social inequality, nutritional quality of some foods or promotion of indiscriminate consumption. Furthermore, treatments for obesity are not well adapted to the bio-psycho-socio peculiarities of obese people and are directed, principally, at modifying so-called lifestyles through disciplined adherence to diets and physical exercise. This vision disregards the fact that health, which is an important motivation for consuming food, is only one of the multiple determinants of daily food intake and does not deal with the fact that eating badly or well may be dressed in different, contradictory or complementary meanings, depending on what is at stake: pleasure, money, eating practices, convenience or illness. The second reason is that this medicalised model bases its strategy for change on providing people with dietary competence and making them responsible for their own health without understanding or at least facing up to the fact that people's daily lives are heterogeneous *per se* and are made up of diverse activities and irregular events which are often incompatible with the routine required by optimum diet.

## Notes

1   In 2000, with the support of the MEC [Ministry of Education and Science] and the Generalitat of Catalunya, I began an ethnographic study in Catalunya (Spain) on the social dimensions of eating disorders and obesity which was part of a broader state-wide programme of research and development on *La alimentación contemporánea desde y más allá de las normas [Contemporary food from the perspective of norms and beyond]*(SEJ2006-15526-Co2 02 PubMed /SOCI). The study, focalised in obesity, has involved three different levels of analysis: a) a review of the studies on the anthropology of food and body, medical anthropology and epidemiological literature, b) an comparative analysis of guidelines on nutritional recommendations and public politics against obesity in Spain, France and Mexico and c) ethnographic work conducted in two specialised clinics on obesity in Catalonia. In this article I only present a critical reflection about the biomedical problematisation of corpulence based mainly on an initial bibliographic review, part of which can be found in Gracia, 2007.

2   The dietary recommendations associated with this diet can be consulted at http://www.msc.es/ciudadanos/proteccion**Salud**/infancia/alimentacion/tema2.htm.

3   The phrases in inverted commas are quotes from other texts. In this case they are from Dapcich, V: Guía de la Alimentación saludable. Madrid: Sociedad Española de Nutrición Comunitaria, 2004, (p. 7).

4 According to the WHO, more than 1,600,000,000 people are overweight and, of those, at least 400,000,000 are obese (http://www.who.int). In Spain, 14.5 % of the adult population is obese and 38.5 % are overweight. The direct and indirect costs associated with this illness are 7 % of total annual health expenditure, that is, about 2,500,000,000 (Strategy for Nutrition, Physical Activity and the Prevention of Obesity. NAOS. Madrid: Spanish Ministry of Health, 2005, p. 9).

5 NAOS, op. cit. pages, 25 and 15 respectively.

6 A more detailed analysis of the relations between biology, history, and culture associated with body weight can be found in Contreras J. and Gracia M. (2005). Op.cit. reference 1.

7 BMI is equal to the individual's weight in kilogrammes divided by the square of their height in metres.

8 NAOS, op.cit p. 11.

9 News published http://www.elpais.com (consulted 27.02.2007) and http://www.deia.com (consulted 2.04.2007).

10 In this article, the authors show the interesting controverse, generated in the US, between anti- and pro-obesity scientists and activists.

11 The explanations on the phenomenon of obesity and the proposal of management vary depending on the theories used by epidemiology. Eclectic and named "eco" approaches are more frequently predominant in the warning and prevention programs (Socorro Parra-Cabrera et al, 1999). For a critical review of the actual epidemiological theories consult Lang and Rayner (2005).

12 NAOS (2005: 21).

13 NAOS (2005: 12).

14 Healthy Guide SENC (2004: 92).

15 NAOS, op. cit. p. 19.

16 NAOS, op. cit. p. 11.

## Bibliography

Alemany, M. (2003). Mecanismes de control del pes corporal. *Revista de la Reial academia de Medicina de Catalunya*, 18, (2): 44-49.

Aranceta, J. (coord). (2002). *Guía Práctica sobre Hábitos de Alimentación y Salud*. Instituto Omega 3, Madrid, SENC.

Aranceta, J. et al. (2005). Prevalencia de obesidad en España. *Med Clin* (Bar), 125 (12): 460-6.

Ascher, F. (2005). *Le mangeur hypermoderne*. Paris: Odile Jacob.

Barquera, S. et al. (2006). *Sobrepeso y obesidad*, Instituto de Salud Pública, México.

Barona, J.L. (2008). Nutrition and Health. The International Context during the Inter-war Crisis. *Social History of Medicine*, vol. 21 (1): 87-105.

Barona, J. L. (2002). *Salud, enfermedad y muerte. La sociedad valenciana entre 1833 y 1939*, Valencia: Institució Alfons El Magnànim.

Basdevant, A. and Guy-Gran, B. (2004). *Médicine de l'obésité.* Paris: Flammarion.

Bolstanki, L. and Thévenot, L. (1991). *De la justification: les économies de la grandeur.* Paris: Gallimard.

Campos, P. (2004). *The Obesity Myth: Why America's Obsession with Weight is Hazardous for your Health.* New York: Gotham Books.

Cheyne, G. (1733). *The English Malady.* London: Strachan.

Contreras, J. and Gracia, M. (eds.) (2004). *La alimentación y sus circunstancias: placer, conveniencia y salud.* Barcelona: IV Foro Internacional de la alimentación.

Conveney, J. (2006). *Food, Morals and Meaning.* London: Routledge.

Crawford, R. (1977). You are dangerous to your health, the ideology of victim blaming. *International Journal of Health Services*, 7, (4): 663-680.

Dapcich, V. et al. (2004). *Guía de la alimentación saludable.* Madrid: Sociedad Española de Nutrición Comunitaria.

De Labarre, M. (2004). Dietética y reflexividad: el "cuidado de sí mismo" contemporáneo. In: Millán, A. (comp.). *Arbitrario cultural. Racionalidad e irracionalidad del comportamiento comensal.* Huesca: La Val de Onsera.

Douglas, M. and Wildawsky, A. (1983). *Risk and culture.* California: University of California Press.

Elias, N. (1989). *El proceso de la civilización.* Madrid: Fondo de Cultura Económica.

Farré, R. (2005). Alimentación y nutrición contemporáneas: realidad y futuro. In Salas Salvadó, J. et al.: *La alimentación y la nutrición a través de la historia.* Barcelona: Editorial Glosa.

Fieldhouse, P. (1996). *Food & nutrition: customs and culture.* London: Chapman & Hall.

Foucault, M. (1989). *Historia de la sexualidad.* Vol. I: *La voluntad de saber.* México D.F.: Siglo XXI Editores.

Gard, M. and Wright, J. (2006). *The obesity epidemic. Science, Morality and Ideology.* London: Routledge.

Generalitat de Catalunya (2005). *Guia l'alimentació saludable a l'etapa escolar.* Barcelona: Generalitat de Catalunya.

Gracia, M. (2004). Thoughts on eating risk and its acceptability. The case of transgenic foods (AGMs). *Brazilian Journal of Nutrition*, 17 (2): 125-149.

Gracia, M. (2007). Comer bien, comer mal: la medicalización del comportamiento alimentario. *Salud Pública de México*, 49 (3): 236-241.

Gracia, M. and Contreras, J. (2008). Corps gros, corps malades? Une perspective socioculturelle. *Corps. Revue Interdisciplinaire*, 4: 63-69.

Lang, T. and Rayner G. (2007). Overcoming policy cacophony on obesity: an ecological public health framework for policymakers. *Obesity Reviews*, 8 (1): 165-181.

Levenstein, H.A. (1996). Diététique contre gastronomie: traditions culinaires, sainteté et santé dans les modèles de vie américains. In: Flandrin, J.L, and M. Montanari, *Histoire de l'alimentation.* Paris: Fayard.

Lupton, D. (2000). Food, risk and subjectivity. In: Williams, S.J. (ed.), *Health, Medicine and Society, Key Theories. Future Agendas.* London: Routledge.

Maddox, G.L. and Liederman, V. (1969). Overweight as a social disability with medical implications. *J. Med Educ* 44: 214-220.

Manzini, I. (1996). L'alimentation et la médecine dans le monde antique. In: Flandrin, J.L., and M. Montanari, *Histoire de l'alimentation*. Paris: Fayard.

Menéndez, L.E. (2002). El malestar actual de la antropología o de la casi imposibilidad de pensar lo ideológico. *Revista de Antropología Social* (11): 39-87.

Mennell, S. (1985). *All manners of food. Eating and Taste in England and France from the Middle Ages to the Present*. Oxford: Basil Blackwell Ltd.

Nestlé, M. (2002). *Food Politics*. Los Angeles: University of California Press.

Parra-Cabrera, S. et al. (1999). Modelos alternativos para el análisis epidemiológico de la obesidad como problema de salud pública. *Revista de Saúde Pública*, 33 (3): 314-325.

Peretti-Watel, P. (2000). *Sociologie du risque*. Paris: Armand Colin.

Pollock, N. (2000). Els àpats i la seva dimensió social (exemples del Sud del Pacífic). *Revista d'Etnologia de Catalunya*, 17: 40-47.

Poulain, J.P. (2000). Les dimensions sociales de l'obésité. In: *Obésité, dépistage et prévention chez l'enfant*. Expertise collective. Paris: INSERM.

Poulain, J.P. (2002). Manger aujourd'hui. Attitudes, normes et pratiques. Toulouse: Éditions Privat.

Powdermaker, H. (1997). An Anthropological Approach to the problem of Obesity. In: Counihan, C. and P. Van Esterik, (eds.), *Food and culture. A reader*. London: Routledge, 370-383.

Ryan, W. (1977). *Blaming the victim*. New York: Vintage Books.

Saguy, A.C. and W.C. Riley (2005). Weighing both sides: morality, mortality, and framing contests over obesity. *Journal of Health Politics, Policy and Law*, 30 (5): 869-921.

Sobal, J. and Stunkard, A.J. (1990). Socioeconomic status and obesity: a review of the literature. *Psychologial Bulletin*, 105: 260-275.

Sobal, J. (1995). The medicalization and demedicalization of obesity. In: Maurer, D. and J. Sobal, (eds): *Eating agendas. Food and nutrition as Social Problems*. New York: Aldine de Gruyter.

Sobal, J. (2001). Commentary: globalization and the epidemiology of obesity, *International Journal of Epidemiology*, 30: 1136-1137.

Tannahill, R. (1988). *Food in History*. London: Penguin Books.

Turner, B.S. (1982). The Government of the Body: Medical Regimens and the Rationalization of Diet. *The British Journal of Sociology*, 33 (2): 254-269.

Turner, B.S. (1999). The discourse of diet. In: Featherstone, M., M. Hepworth, and B. Turner, (eds.), *The Body. Social Process and Cultural Theory*. London: Sage Publications.

Vigarello, G. (2006). *Lo sano y lo malsano*. Madrid, Abadía Lectores.

World Health Organization (2004). *57ª Asamblea Mundial de la Salud. Estrategia Mundial sobre régimen alimentario, actividad física y salud*. In: www.who.int/gb/ebwha/pdf_files/WHA57/A57_R17-sp.pdf.

Caterina Masana Bofarull

Chapter XII.

# Self-care and management of adults with chronic illness and dependency: The Spanish case in the context of the new Dependency Law*

## Introduction

The ever-increasing number of chronic illnesses that create dependency has become a challenge for developed countries. The problem lies in precisely how to articulate self-care (by sick persons and their social networks) and the management of illness through health and social policy. The present situation in Spain reveals the limitations of both self-care and policy solutions – despite recently implemented legislation (*Dependency Law*) – in responding to the challenge of chronicity and dependency, which requires long-term care. There are two main reasons why this is the case, and these are the subject of this chapter.

First, in Spain care for the chronically ill is still considered a private matter to be handled by the family through what is known as 'informal support', a fact that reveals the limitations of the public healthcare system. This model is unsustainable even in the short term, as a consequence of important social and demographic changes and shifting roles within the family.

Second, the Spanish healthcare system and social services are structured in a way that prevents coordinated care provision. The powers of various administrative bodies at the level of the state and in the 17 autonomous communities[1] overlap and conflict both with each other and with private services. The order of priorities is based on a biomedical understanding of health, sickness and care subject to political and economical constraints and operating on a limited budget without taking into consideration the voices of those affected.

This chapter is an attempt to show that an interdisciplinary approach based on collaboration between biomedicine and the social sciences (in particular medical anthropology) is needed to help formulate the health and social policies required to meet this new challenge.

## Chronicity and dependency: a new challenge for the 21st century

The steady increase in recent years of chronic illnesses leading to loss of independence constitutes both a health problem and a social problem. Until the 1960s, acute infectious diseases were the primary focus of the publicly funded healthcare system because of their high rate of morbidity and mortality. However, advances in medical science, technology and public health (such as immunisations, sanitation, housing and education) have contributed to a decrease in those acute diseases. As a result, life expectancy has risen during this period. From a biomedical point of view, longer life expectancy – in addition to other factors such as bad habits concerning diet, physical activity, the consumption of noxious substances, such as tobacco, etc. – increases individual risk of chronic illness.[2]

At present, chronic diseases account for more than half the world's morbidity rate: i.e. 60 per cent of the 58 million deaths in 2005 (WHO, 2006). Because of this, chronic diseases (mainly those that lead to dependence) are the new challenge for the health and social policies of developed countries with a welfare state (such as Spain), and they are considered by many to constitute a worldwide epidemic (WHO, 2005).[3]

## Chronicity and dependency: assessment and definition

A chronic disease is defined as an organic or functional disorder that persists for a long period of time, and is characterised by gradual onset and an uncertain prognosis; in principle, there is no cure (Nobel, 1991).[4] Individuals in all age groups may be affected, although adults and the elderly predominate (Avellaneda, 2006). The wide variety of disorders involved makes chronic diseases difficult to classify. There are several commonly accepted classifications using different criteria based on: 1) Frequency or prevalence (i.e., common vs. rare diseases); 2) Whether or not they generate disability; 3) Prognosis (bad, uncertain, or good); and 4) The degree of dependency they generate (moderate, severe or total). Additional criteria include the presence or absence of pain, a sense of loss or physical threat, and changes in or loss of body image. Finally, chronic diseases are also classified on the basis of specialised fields of medicine: cardiovascular, respiratory, metabolic and endocrinological, musculoskeletal, neurological, and so on.

These classifications, however useful, have their limitations, since the course of chronic illnesses is neither as unidirectional nor as 'natural' as we have been led to suppose (Kleinman, 2000). Expected outcomes do not always materialise, especially given the complexity and heterogeneity of both chronic diseases and individual biology. Diagnosis and classification return us to the problem of taking a strictly biological view that excludes the social and cultural aspects of illness (Menéndez, 1978). It is not a question of denying the physiopathological reality of chronic diseases, but of recognising the importance of cultural context and the *social* course of the illness (Kleinman, 2000).

Beyond this, however, chronic diseases create a significant disturbance in people's lives that causes them to modify their lifestyles to readjust to the new constraints resulting from the disease. This is especially relevant in the case of illnesses that generate disability and/or dependency. The need to modify one's lifestyle in order to adjust to new limitations affects not only sick persons but those around them, especially those who are their primary caregivers.

In Spain, dependency is legally defined in the *Dependency Law* as:

> The permanent condition of persons who, because of a lack of, or decrease in, physical, intellectual or sensorial autonomy, require the assistance of one or more persons or require important assistance to carry out the basic activities of daily life.[5]

The law classifies three degrees of dependency (lesser to greater): moderate, severe, and total dependency (in Spanish, *gran dependencia*) including two levels within these degrees. The current definition of dependency centers on two aspects: 1) The ability to carry out what have been called the 'Basic Activities of Daily Life',[6] as opposed to the earlier definition based on 'normal' anatomy and physiology. 2) Adaptation to one's surroundings, which implies greater or lesser dependence on assistance from others.[7]

The legal definition and assessment of dependency may seem straightforward, but in practice it is problematic. Persons who wish to receive services or benefits from the new law must have their degree of dependence evaluated. The official criteria used to evaluate dependency[8] are both highly restrictive and applied in a way that excludes a significant number of persons, who will not be able to benefit from any service because they are not considered dependent (regardless of whether they are or not).

The universal coverage and equal access on which the law is based is thus compromised. However, the voices of those affected have raised a claim for re-evaluation.[9]

## Chronicity and dependency care needs: long-term care (LTC)

Long-term care (LTC), specifically for chronic diseases that create dependency (henceforth, CDD),[10] refers to the provision of services for persons with long-term functional dependency, regardless of age. Chronicity together with dependency creates the need for a range of services. The World Health Organization points to the following consequences of a chronic disease (WHO, 2003:247): limited capacity to carry out the activities of daily living; difficulties in accessing healthcare and complying with healthcare regimes; diminished ability of the individual to maintain a healthy lifestyle and to prevent deterioration in health and functional status; additional emotional needs and strains; and social needs that arise from limitations on maintaining regular social contacts.[11]

In Spain, the expression used to refer to the concept of long-term care (LTC) is *atención sociosanitaria*, which can be translated as *sociomedical care*. This expression first appeared in Catalonia[12] in a ministerial order regulating an integrated and permanent LTC service provided by the public social services and health services for people with chronic diseases, the elderly and other groups without specific regulation. The Spanish state later redefined the concept of *atención sociosanitaria* as:

> ... all forms of care provided for patients, many of whom are chronically ill, who can benefit from simultaneous and synergic provision of health and social services to improve their autonomy, remove limitations, relieve suffering and return them to full membership in society.[13]

While these intentions are laudable, they are often not realised in practice.

## Self-care in adults with chronic diseases and dependency

In Spain, 88 % of chronic care is provided by the patient's social network, mainly close relatives (a role that falls almost exclusively to women).[14] This fact exposes the limitations of sociomedical coverage provided by the state. These so-called 'informal'[15] care practices or 'informal support' have been analysed using a wide variety of different terms that bring particular dimensions into focus (i.e., domestic medicine, home care, self-help and others; see Haro 2000 for a detailed comparison and analysis of terms).

Following Menéndez (2003), I have preferred to use the analytic category of self-care, understood as 'beliefs and practices used by individuals and groups to explain, care, control, relieve, endure, cure, resolve or prevent processes that affect their health…without central, direct, and intentional intervention by the healthcare professionals, even though they may be the frame of reference for these activities' (Menéndez 2003:198). As well as self-care understood as 'an attempt by sick persons and their families and social networks to take control of the care process through practices' following Illich's categorisation of appropriation of health (Illich, 1975), self-care is an umbrella category that subsumes the others, and includes all practices (medical, logistical, emotional/social) both within the home and outside it. These constitute the first level of care, the very first step taken in response to a health problem. An analytic focus on these practices allows us to address the question of agency. The chronically ill and dependent, and their families and social networks, are not simply passive receivers of services provided by the state, but active interpreters of their situation and their needs. Anthropology of medicine should recognise that primary healthcare takes place outside clinical contexts, and be attentive not only to the macro-level effects of health policies on populations, but to their micro-level impacts on and interactions with individual lives.

## Care practices and levels of care provision

The hegemonic biomedical model distinguishes between two levels of care provision: medical and sociomedical care. Care practices may be oriented either towards cure or towards care. Curative medical care has been at the center of the biomedical model for decades, and it has proved successful in treating acute diseases. Chronic diseases, however, challenge this model because in many cases cure is elusive (Comelles, 1988). Dependency and the need for long-term care require a different model: sociomedical care. The error of the curative model is the assumption that medical care ends after the patient is discharged from the hospital or leaves the doctor's office.[16] At this point, when the patient either begins the process of recovery or starts learning to live with the illness, the medical system largely withdraws, leaving the responsibility for both medical care and caregiving to the sick persons and their families. The new *Dependency Law* is an attempt by the state to address this situation and to recognise the importance of caregiving. The law recognises practices that support personal hygiene, shopping, preparation of meals, housekeeping, mobility within the home, and other 'Basic Activities of Daily Life', but these fall far short of meeting the needs of persons living with chronic illness and dependency.

An anthropologically informed approach to the study of self-care needs and practices examines the contradictions, dissonances and paradoxes that arise at different levels of care. The analytic model proposed here identifies three levels: medical care, logistical support, and emotional/social support. *Medical care* refers to the personal care of the ill person in terms of the basic and/or instrumental needs most related to health: personal hygiene, nutrition, administration of medication and/or other treatments. *Logistical support* involves assistance related to needs such as housekeeping (cleaning, food shopping, etc.) but also other activities outside the domestic context such accompanying the sick person to medical appointments or tests and helping with other personal tasks. *Emotional/social support* includes a wide variety of possibilities depending on the personal relationship between the ill person and the relative or friend: talking, listening, going for a walk, or other recreational and social activities.

## First level: medical care

A chronically ill person's therapeutic itinerary within the public healthcare system generally begins in one of two ways. One possibility is that the person feels unwell and goes to the primary healthcare clinic. Following a lengthy series of visits and tests, if the primary care physician suspects a particular diagnosis, the patient is referred to a specialist who then takes charge of the case. Alternatively, the patient may have an accident or experience an acute health problem requiring hospitalisation. In both cases, once diagnosed with a chronic disease and/or discharged from the hospital, the patient will periodically see the specialist (for relapses, worsening of symptoms or follow-up) and/or the primary care physician (in some cases for follow-up, but in most to obtain prescriptions for medications).

At this level of care, the above-mentioned classification of chronic diseases by medical specialty gives rise to certain problems. First, the patient's disorder may fall within more than one specialty. As a result, the patient is shuttled from one specialist to another and is repeatedly scheduled for more diagnostic tests, a process that delays diagnosis and treatment. Second, not all primary care physicians are sufficiently prepared or experienced to handle the variety and complexity of chronic diseases,[17] nor do they have administrative authorisation to order more specialised diagnostic tests. Third, waiting lists for both appointments with specialists and diagnostic tests delays needed treatment. Finally, in cases of comorbidity, specialists treating the same patient often fail to share information with each other or coordinate treatment plans, with the result that adverse drug interactions may occur, and diagnostic and follow-up tests that could be scheduled together are scheduled separately. The patient's time and energy is wasted in unnecessary trips, waiting lists lengthen into weeks and even months, and healthcare costs rise.

Additionally, in Spain, a private medical care system coexists with the public system. Private insurance companies play an increasingly important role in making up for the deficits of the public system. They can provide complementary services concerning those not included in the public system (like dental care and unconventional treatments), as well as supplementary services that increase individual choice with regard to the providers of these services, thus facilitating an easier and quicker access to medical services – mainly to avoid waiting lists (López-Casasnovas, 2007). The main question concerning the private insurance, is the unequal access to services for those without economic means to face the costs of it. People with CDD who cannot afford a private insurance are at a greater disadvantage in this dual system[18] than the rest of the population. They may require special long-term care services, and in any case they are more frequent users of medical services, spending a much greater proportion of their time in waiting rooms and on waiting lists. In consequence, if they cannot afford a private insurance, they must rely on the public healthcare system whose limitations can directly affect the illness process, in some cases leading to not desired iatrogenic[19] problems.

In Spain, in addition to the public and private medical care systems, chronically ill persons often have recourse to various forms of complementary and/or alternative medicine[20] – such as traditional Chinese medicine and homeopathy – to relieve symptoms that remain frustratingly resistant to standard biomedical treatments. Though the existence of medical pluralism suggests the advantages of a greater range of choice, the reality shows us the difficulties and inequality in accessing the services, again due to economic reasons, because most of these services are not covered by the public healthcare system.[21]

Independently, however, of whether the chronically ill seek medical attention through the private system, the public system, or CAM, with very few exceptions – for example those receiving outpatient treatment or benefiting from the services of a visiting nurse – the first level of medical care (i.e. personal hygiene, nutrition, administration of medication, nursing care, etc.) is self-care provided in the domestic realm by the patients themselves and by their caregivers,[22] who are identified, paradoxically and unfairly, as 'informal support'.

At this point, it is necessary to understand the political structure[23] of health and social services in Spain, which is rather fragmented. Health services are provided through the Spanish Ministry of Health and Social Policy and corresponding departments of health in the autonomous communities. Social services, however, are mainly provided (except for dependency issues) through the Ministry of Labour and Immigration and corresponding departments of social welfare in the autonomous communities[24]. The existence of these two ('four') different administrative levels helps to explain the lack of coordinated care for the chronically ill and dependent, and other bureaucratic complications that arise when there is a need for both medical and sociomedical services. For example, a specialist may decide that the patient requires home care by a visiting nurse on a daily basis, but when the patient leaves the doctor's office, he or she must then request this through the social services bureaucracy. This places an additional burden on chronically ill persons and their families or caregivers who must use time and energy because of the public administration bureaucracy, which could otherwise be unified and streamlined through coordination between health and social services.

## Second level: logistical support

The logistical needs of the chronically ill proposed here are not limited to housekeeping (cleaning, food shopping, etc.) but include activities outside the domestic context such as assistance in scheduling and keeping appointments for medical visits and tests, and helping with other personal tasks. It has taken many years for some of these needs to be recognised. They have been rendered invisible by relegating care for the chronically ill to the family as a private matter. This approach, given social and demographic changes in Spanish society, is unsustainable even in the short term. The Spanish state's *Dependency White Paper* (2004:33, 73),[25] points out that 'there are fewer adult women available as caregivers, and more persons in need of long-term care' (among other reasons). But, it is not that there are fewer women, it is (as they also recognise) that many women have responsibilities outside the home. Women have entered the labour force in large numbers, and their role within the family has changed. As a result of the difficulty of balancing the competing demands of work and family, they have less time to assume the role of caregivers as was traditionally the case.[26]

In addition, the increase in the proportion of elderly persons in the population means that there are more dependent persons, and workplace and traffic accidents also increase the number of dependent people of all ages. Moreover, family structures are going through other important changes. The traditional domestic model of the extended family is disappearing with increasing geographic mobility and distance between family members, leading to an increase in the variety of family models and domestic units (more people live alone or as a couple).

These social and demographic changes are fundamental to an analysis of the impact of private caregiving practices and public policies on care of the chronically ill and dependent, because they reconfigure the demands made by families on the healthcare system (Duran, 2004; Comas d'Argemir, 2007). Many families appear to be unable (and in some cases unwilling)[27] to assume the role of caregivers as they did in the past. Families demand public policies, which take responsibility for and respond to the care needs. As taxpayers whose money funds the public healthcare system, citizens demand the right to be looked after.

It is in this context that the *Dependency Law*[28] was devised as an attempt to resolve the problem of managing the care of the chronically ill and dependent, and relieving the burden on their families. The main aim of this law is to guarantee access to sociomedical services and/or economic benefits for those persons in a situation of dependency. While at first glance this new law seems to be an adequate response to the care needs of those affected, a more careful analysis, however, reveals certain weaknesses and problems.

Long-term care needs imply a considerable increase in public health expenditure as a result of increased social demand. Care of dependent persons increases sociomedical expenses tenfold (mainly because of chronic diseases), and constitutes an estimated 75 % of health expenses and 80 % of pharmaceutical expenses in developed countries (García-Sarriá, 2005: 16). The new law arrives at a time of economic crisis, underfunding of public services in general, and the need to contain rising healthcare costs, and its brief history suggests that the state will not be able to maintain and provide the promised services and benefits at desired levels.[29] Many families who applied for benefits under the law are still waiting, months later, for these benefits to materialise. Many others will not be able to receive any benefit, because the law establishes a personal means test: i.e. beyond a certain income level, people lose the right to claim benefits regardless of their degree of dependency. This suggests the loss of universal coverage and equal access on which the law is based. Moreover, the order of priorities is based on a biomedical understanding of health, sickness and care, subject to economical and political rationality and constraints, and operating on a limited budget, without considering the values, opinions, needs and preferences of the public (Sanz, 2005).

Because the family caregiver of a person with CDD cannot work full-time outside the home, and because caring for someone with CDD involves increased domestic expenses (Duran, 1999), the law makes possible a so-called salary for the family caregiver, but only under exceptional circumstances, and requires the caregiver to undergo training.[30] As far as I am concerned, this aspect of the law seems aimed at professionalising domestic care: on the one hand, relegating it to professionals who were previously required to be authorised – thus further perpetuating the biomedical and hegemonic way of providing care and, on the other, professionalising contractually the family caregivers. This raises social and ethical questions that medical anthropology is well positioned to address. Is the ideal relationship between chronically ill persons and their caregivers primarily professional rather than affective? How will this affect the relationship between trained and 'professionalised' family caregivers and their sick relatives?

Finally, the implementation of the law together with the creation of the National Dependency System (SND),[31] as the fourth pillar of the welfare state, involves the creation of a new macrostructure of authorised institutions to deal with the dependency issue. This new organigram, however, does not resolve the problem of conflicting powers held by the health or social service departments at different administrative levels, because even though it is designed to be an independent fourth support of the welfare state, it is in fact dependent on the bureaucracies of the health and social services, at both the ministerial and the autonomous community level, thus making coordination even more complicated.

## Third level: emotional/social support

The emotional and social needs of the chronically ill and dependent are especially relevant because they are not addressed by the strictly medical and sociomedical services provided by the state, and because they are directly related to self-care. Seen from an anthropological perspective, this third level of care proposed here is based on the understanding that social and emotional support constitutes a form of care because family and social networks are a key factor in the psychological and emotional health of sick persons (Kleinman, 2000; Canals, 2002). Limiting the definition of caregivers to those who help the chronically ill to cope with material, instrumental or logistical problems blinds us to the sick person's other needs. If the aim is to achieve a better quality of life for people by responding further to biological or social needs, the emotional and affective ones should also be taken into consideration (Carrasco, 2003).

The World Health Organization in its long-term care policy document (WHO, 2003) recommends paying attention to emotional and social needs: 'Dependency creates additional emotional needs and strains which must also be addressed. Social needs also arise from limitations in maintaining regular social contacts'. However, this emotional/social support level seems to be quite 'invisible' in Spanish sociomedical policy, including the *Dependency Law*, although it makes use of the concept of biopsychosocial care,[32] and despite the *Dependency White Paper* (on which the Law is based) specifically refers to this kind of support.

*The Dependency White Paper* (2004) mentions emotional support in connection with intergenerational relationships between chronically ill grandparents and their grandchildren,[33] and the need for family caregivers to receive emotional support through mutual help groups.[34] Sick persons are said to benefit from a 'form of help that persons receive from their social networks', (op.cit. 2004:172) categorised into emotional support (of an affective nature), informational and strategic support (help in solving problems), and material or instrumental support (such as all care practices for dependent persons). Emotional/social support does not, however, constitute a central theme in the sociomedical care of the chronically ill and dependent. It just appears in the chapter on long-term care by family caregivers when conceptualising 'informal support', where the general point of view of the professionals who drafted it (mainly social psychologists) are in favour of maintaining and even expanding the 'informal support' model.

While a social worker can never replace the emotional/social support that the sick person should receive from a family member or friend, we should also remember that the responsibility for providing this kind of support for a chronically ill and dependent family member carries a heavy moral charge in Spanish society, and this engenders ambivalent feelings in those on whom this responsibility falls. While they want to help those they love, they also feel the strain of combining these tasks with their personal and working lives. (op.cit. 2004:217). The first approach to the study of care practices shows, paradoxically, that in Spain – a country which traditionally has relied on the 'informal care' model – the self-care model can also be deficient or inadequate, thus revealing the limitations of family caregivers to cope with the burden of caring for chronic and dependent relatives.[35] *The Dependency White Paper* (2004: 172) points out that 'having a large social network of family and friends is not, in and of itself, a guarantee of sufficient help and support in the event of need for prolonged or permanent care'.

The holistic perspective of anthropology shows us that illness processes are a social experience (Kleinman, 2000; Kleinman, 1980; Comelles, 1998) and a cultural phenomenon (Kleinman, 1980; Comelles and Martínez, 1993; Comelles and Perdiguero, 2000) located not only in the individual body as an embodied human agency (Merleau-Ponty, 1993, Bourdieu, 1977) but in the sick person's life world (*lebenswelt*) (Husserl, 1991), and affecting everyone in it. For these reasons, and for a deeper analysis of care practices, I suggest here investigating further the concept of care/assistance/attention, understood as limited to functional activities or tasks. Considering that 'to take care' of someone means to 'care about' someone, I propose to look also at care in terms of attitude and interaction between the sick person and the social network (caregivers or otherwise), understood as an intersubjective nature of social life (Goffman, 1989).[36] Individuals live in an intersubjective world of social commitments, and thus, the needs of the sick persons and the demands they place on their families or social networks must be in concordance with the nature of those personal relationships (Kleinman, 1987). Caring for sick relatives is a commitment that reflects the concept of reciprocity (Mauss, 1991; Canals; 2002), with social rules and implicit or explicit agreements based on an updated concept of community, the arena where 'informal' care takes place. The essence of this third level of care may be summarised as follows:

> The most traditional form of healthcare consisted of sleeping, eating, loving, working, playing, dreaming, singing, and suffering…and curing was a traditional way of consoling, caring for, comforting, accepting, tolerating, and also rejecting the afflicted.[37]

## Conclusions

People with chronic diseases and dependency require long-term care services that are not yet sufficiently guaranteed by the Spanish state's public healthcare and social services system – despite the recently implemented *Dependency Law* – and this places a serious burden on the families of sick persons. Social and demographic changes make it impossible to continue providing this care through 'informal support' as has been done up to now.

Part of the role of an applied anthropology of medicine is, through the analysis of public policy in regard to health, to promote open discussion of social problems between civil society and public administration in order to contribute to resolving them (Singer and Castro, 2004: xiii). The ethnographically informed critique of policy, the use of ethnographic data to increase the effectiveness of existing policies, to assist in the drafting of new policy, and, most recently, to identify weaknesses and unintended negative consequences of policy on people's lives and well-being, as I have tried to do in this chapter, are all ways in which a 'public-interest anthropology' (Singer and Castro 2004, xii) can contribute to the public debate.

The current increase in the proportion of the adult population with chronic diseases and dependency in Spain represents a public health and policy issue with multiple social, economic and political implications. One of the contributions of anthropology is to show that many different forces shape health policies, only one of which is concern for the public health. In this chapter I have tried to suggest what some of these forces are in the Spanish case, and to show the kinds of impact they have on the lives of chronically ill and dependent persons.

A structural change in beliefs, practices and priorities concerning processes of health, sickness and care is necessary in order to arrive at policy solutions that combine the advantages of self-care with those of the welfare state. A public-interest medical anthropology is especially well positioned to provide the arguments, based on empirical evidence, for a redesign of healthcare priorities and policies in concert with health professionals, policy makers, and those affected by chronic illness and dependency.

## Notes

\*   Translation: Susan M. DiGiacomo, PhD.

1   Following the end of the Franco dictatorship in 1975, during the transition to democracy over the late 1970s and early 1980s the Spanish state was restructured into 17 autonomous communities, each with a somewhat different political and fiscal relationship to the state, and a distinctive range of home-rule powers that include healthcare, social services, and education. This new structure was superimposed upon but did not replace the earlier territorial division of Spain into 50 provinces, a structure copied from the French state early in the 19th century.

2 Although the origins of chronic diseases are complex, *risk* is defined here as "a probability of an adverse outcome, or a factor that raises this probability" (WHO, 2002:10).

3 Chronic diseases are also a problem in developing countries, not just developed ones, although this subject is beyond the scope of this paper.

4 Cited in Avellaneda (2006) and Avellaneda et al. (2007).

5 Law 39/2006 (known as the *Dependency Law*): Preliminary Title, Article 2.2, BOE 299:44144.

6 In Spanish, *Actividades Básicas de la Vida Diaria (ABVD)* are defined in the *Dependency Law* as activities essential for living independently, for which the standards are established in the Evaluation Criteria for Situations of Dependency (Law 39/2006. Preliminary Title, Article 2.3., BOE 299:44144). To these have been added Instrumental Activities of Daily Life (AIVD – *Actividades Instrumentales de la Vida Diaria*), which are more complex and presuppose a greater degree of personal autonomy (the cognitive and motor abilities to manage everyday tasks), as specified in the *Dependency White Paper* (2004:36).

7 Other classifications have also been proposed concerning different kinds of dependency. Avellaneda (2006) employs a four-part classificatory scheme: physical, mental or cognitive, social and economic.

8 In Spanish, *Baremo de Valoración de la Situación de Dependencia* (BVSD). Published in the BOE (Boletín Oficial del Estado, the Spanish state's official record in which new legislation is published) Núm.96 21/04/2007.

9 Patients' associations and other organisations and institutions (public and private) point out that these criteria fail to meet the complex needs of many persons affected by chronic diseases and dependency. For example, the Spanish Neuropsychiatry Association (Asociación Española de Neuropsiquiatría, AEN) has argued, with some success, that somatic criteria should not be used to define disabilities and dependency resulting from mental illness. *Valoración de la AEN sobre el Baremo de Valoración de la Situación de Dependencia*, available at: http://www.aen.es/web/docs/AENyLeyDepen07.pdf [accessed June 11, 2009]

10 The abbreviation CDD is used throughout this paper to refer to chronic diseases and dependency.

11 These emotional and social needs will be discussed in a later section of this chapter.

12 Catalonia is one of the above mentioned autonomous communities (see footnote 1). Ministerial order for the creation of the program '*Living longer, living better': sociomedical care for elders with LTC diseases. ("Vida als anys" d'atenció sòcio-sanitària a la gent gran amb llarga malaltia*. ORDRE 29-05-1986, DOGC núm. 694, June 2, 1986).

13 Law 16/2003, Chapter I, Article 14, page 20573. Law of *Cohesión y Calidad del Sistema Nacional de Salud* [Cohesion and Quality of the National Health Care System], approved 28 May 2003.

14 Aguirre (2005); Avellaneda, A. (2006); Avellaneda et al. (2007); Duran, M.A. (1999, 2004); Garcia-Calvente, M.M. et al. (1999).

15 The quotation marks are deliberate because I disagree with the implications of this word, although a discussion of the differences between professional and informal (lay or non-professional) knowledge is beyond the scope of this article.

16 Hospitalisation does not, however, necessarily precede long-term care. Many chronically ill persons have never been hospitalised.

17 The question of physician competence in treating chronic diseases is beyond the scope of this chapter. In this regard, however, a 2005 WHO publication *Preparación de los profesionales de la atención de salud para el siglo XXI. El reto de las enfermedades crónicas* stresses the importance of preparing health professionals for the demands of the transition from treating acute problems to treating chronic diseases, and proposes broadening the qualifications of medical personnel in the following respects: 1) Patient-centered care; 2) Cooperation and communication both with patients and other health professionals; 3) Safety and quality of healthcare; 4) Use of information technology to improve patient follow-up and information sharing between physicians; and 5) Continuity of patient care.

18 Possibility of combining public health system and private health insurance.

19 I use this concept here in the same clinical/structural sense as Illich (1975).

20 There is still no consensus about how to categorise these healing practices of unconventional medicine, although *Complementary and Alternative Medicine* (abbreviated as CAM) is the most widely accepted terminology (Perdiguero, 2004:141).

21 The Catalan government's department of health is currently studying the possibility of public coverage of some forms of alternative and complementary medicine, such as homeopathy, following the example of Holland, although it remains to be seen whether this will come to pass. While a very few primary healthcare centres and hospitals in Catalonia include these treatments, the cost is borne by the patient.

22 The social workers I have interviewed in Catalonia who are in direct contact with caregivers commented favourably on the quality of care provided by family members, although they also note that in some cases, and in some areas such as hygiene and nursing care, they require more training and professional support.

23 The organisational structure of the public healthcare system in Spain is tax-based and administratively decentralised. While the state retains the legislative and regulatory power to establish minimum standards and requirements for medical and sociomedical care provision, the governments of the 17 autonomous communities decide how to organise and provide services.

24 Since June 2009 the names of the state's ministries have changed, which has also meant some change in the structure. The former Ministry of Health and Social Policy is now named the Ministry of Health and Consumer Affairs. The Ministry of Labour and Immigration is now known as the Ministry of Labour and Social Affairs. The National Dependence System, which came under the Ministry of Labour, is now under the Ministry of Health. Moreover, social services are provided through both Ministries, thus making coordination more confusing. At the autonomous community level, such as Catalonia, health and social departments have not changed their names or their structure up to now, but dependency issues come under the Social Department (which is the opposite of the state ministry, where dependency issues come under the Health Ministry).

25 The *Dependency Law* is based on a previous technical report, the *Dependency White Paper* (*Libro Blanco de la Dependencia en España*, 2004), which contains information from several studies (mainly in sociology, economics and psychology) concerning dependency in Spain.

26 This is not a problem limited to those caring for a chronically ill and dependent family member. The difficulty of combining work and family obligations is a current problem for many Spanish families and a subject of social and political debate. Aguirre (2005); Duran (1999).

27 Caring for sick relatives is inextricably linked to morality, the moral duty of assisting those in need. Sickness is a moral experience to which caregiving is a moral response (moral acts); see Kleinman and Benson (2004).

28 The complete name of the law is *Law for the promotion of personal autonomy and care for persons in a situation of dependency* (*Ley de promoción de la autonomía personal y atención a las personas en situación de dependencia*) Law 39/2006, 14 December. The Spanish Parliament approved it on 30 November 2006, to come into effect on 1 January 2007. For understandable reasons, it is referred to simply as the *Dependency Law* (*Ley de Dependencia*).

29 The *Dependency Law* is insufficient funded by the central government. As a result, the governments of the autonomous communities, which are responsible for applying the law, must cope with the new costs created from the new services offered by the state's law. Both lack the resources to apply it.

30 Under the law, the family caregiver will have contractual rights and obligations. The state will decide when he or she can take days off or vacations, and when he/she must attend training courses.

31 The National Dependency System – *Sistema Nacional de Dependencia, SND* creates the System for Autonomy and Attention of Dependency organism (SAAD – *Sistema para la Autonomía y Atención a la Dependencia*) –whose aim is "a coordinated system of services and benefits, for the prevention, care and protection of persons, through a coordinated network of public and private (previously authorised) institutions and services, with the cooperation of all Public Administrations" (i.e., the Spanish state and the governments of the autonomous communities) (*Dependency Law* 39/2006, Title I, Chapter I, Article 6, BOE 299: 44146).

32 Only, however, in reference to day or night care centres or residential centres: 'Residential care based on a biopsychosocial approach, provides continuing services of a personal and medical nature' (*Dependency Law* 39/2006, Title I, Chapter II, Article 25, BOE 299:44149). The law does not specify what these 'personal' services consist of.

33 '...this intergenerational relationship constitutes an incalculable and irreplaceable source of emotional support both for children and for the elderly.' (Dependency White Paper, 2004: 183).

34 Mutual help groups (in Spanish, *grupos de ayuda mútua*, abbreviated to GAM) of people affected by a specific disease are part of health/support associations for those affected (in Spanish, AA, *asociaciones de afectados* or AS, *asociaciones de salud*) and other entities known as the 'third sector'. Although these groups and associations implicitly accept the biomedical paradigm, they attempt to fill mainly emotional/social needs not addressed by either medical institutions or by patients' social networks (Canals, 2003). 'These groups act as providers and receivers of emotional support by allowing for the expression of feelings and opinions and to identify oneself in a group of equals.' (Dependency White Paper, 2004:390).

35 Emotional or social support is not only necessary for the chronically ill and dependent persons, but for their family caregivers, who bear a significant emotional burden. However, this aspect is beyond the scope of this chapter.

36  From an epistemological and phenomenological perspective (see Taylor, Husserl, Dilthey, Merleau-Ponty, Heidegger, Wittgenstein) and to the relations between sick persons and 'healthy' ones, from a symbolic interaction perspective (see Goffman, 1989; Parsons, 1999; Becker, 1964).

37  Illich (1975:116), citing Gubser, A (1967) and Sigerist, H.E. (1967). My translation.

## Bibliography

Avellaneda, A. (2006). Atención Sociosanitaria en las Enfermedades Raras. Un modelo para las enfermedades crónicas discapacitantes [Sociomedical Care for Rare Diseases. A model for chronic diseases that create disability]. Unpublished doctoral dissertation, Universidad Rey Juan Carlos, Madrid.

Avellaneda, A., Izquierdo, M., Torrent-Farnell, J. and Ramón, J.R. (2007). Enfermedades raras: enfermedades crónicas que requieren un nuevo enfoque sociosanitario [Rare Diseases: chronic diseases that need a new approach]. *Anales Sistema Sanitario Navarra*, Vol. 30 (2), mayo-agosto, 177-190.

Aguirre, R. (2005). *Los cuidados familiares como problema público y objeto de políticas [Family care as a public problem and a political issue]* Ponencia presentada en CEPAL Reunión de Expertos: *Políticas hacia las familias, protección e inclusión sociales*.

Becker, H. (1964). *Los extraños. Sociología de la desviación [Outsiders. Studies in the Sociology of deviance]*. Buenos Aires: Tiempo Contemporáneo.

Bourdieu, P. (1977). *The Anthropology of the Body*. New York: Academic Press.

Canals, J. (2002). *El regreso de la reciprocidad. Grupos de ayuda mutua y asociaciones de personas afectadas en la crisis del Estado del Bienestar [The return of reciprocity. Mutual help groups and associations of affected persons in the welfare state crisis]*. Doctoral dissertation. Universitat Rovira i Virgili, Departament d'Antropologia, Filosofia i Treball Social. Tarragona.

Canals, J. (2003). Grupos de ayuda mutua y asociaciones de personas afectadas: Reciprocidades, identidades y dependencias [Mutual help groups and patient support associations: reciprocity, identity and dependency]. In: Filgueira, J. and López-Fernández, I. (eds.), *Antropología y Salud Mental*. Cuadernos de Psiquiatría Comunitaria. Vol. 3, (1): 71-81. Available at: http://www.aen.es/aAW/web/cas/publicaciones/Otros/index.jsp [accessed June 11, 2009]

Carrasco, C. (2003). *El cuidado: ¿coste o prioridad social? [Care: cost or social priority?]*. Ponencia presentada en el Congreso Internacional Sare 2003. *Cuidar cuesta: costes y beneficios del cuidado*. [Care costs: the costs and benefits of care] Gastéiz: Emakunde-Instituto Vasco de la Mujer y Comunidad Europea / Fondo Social Europeo.

Comas d'Argemir, D. (2007). Dependència vs. Autonomia. Família i politiques públiques en l'assistència i cura de les persones [Dependency vs. autonomy. Family and public policy concerning healthcare and personal care]. Paper presented at the VI Jornada de Treball Social de la URV, 17 May 2007.

Comelles, J.M. (1988). *Acerca de la construcción sociocultural de la cronicidad [About socio-cultural construction of chronicity].* In: *Jano*, Vol. XXXIV (808): 43-49.

Comelles, J.M. and Martínez, A. (1993). *Enfermedad, cultura y sociedad [Illness, culture and society].* Madrid: Eudema.

Comelles, J.M. (1996). *El papel del sistema de salud en la configuración de la demanda de servicios [The role of the health system in the shaping of demand for services].* In: AA.VV. *El usuario como determinante de la oferta de servicios sanitarios [Users as determinants of medical services offered].* Madrid, Comunidad de Madrid, Consejería de Salud, Dirección General de Planificación, Formación e Investigación,.29-41.

Comelles, J.M. (1998). Sociedad, salud y enfermedad: los procesos asistenciales [Society, health and sickness: processes of care]. *Trabajo Social y Salud*, 29: 135-150.

Comelles, J.M. and Perdiguero, E. (2000). *Medicina y Cultura. Estudios entre la Antropología y la Medicina [Medicine and culture. Essays in the borderland between anthropology and medicine].* Barcelona: Bellaterra.

*Dependency White Paper. Care for people in a situation of dependency in Spain* (2004). Ministry of Labor and Social Affairs. *Libro Blanco de la Dependencia. Atención a las personas en situación de dependencia en España.* Ministerio de Trabajo y Asuntos Sociales, December 2004. Available at: http://www.tt.mtas.es/periodico/serviciossociales/200501/libro_blanco_dependencia.htm [accessed June 23 2009]

Durán, M.A. (1999). *Costes invisibles de la enfermedad [The invisible costs of sickness].* Bilbao: Fundación BBVA.

Durán, M.A. (2004). *Las demandas sanitarias de las familias [Demand for healthcare from families].*

Gaceta Sanitaria; 18 (1): 195-200.

García-Calvente, M.M.; Mateo-Rodríguez, I. and Gutiérrez, P. (1999). *Cuidados y cuidadores en el sistema informal de salud [Care practices and caregivers in the informal health system].* Granada: Escuela Andaluza de Salud Pública.

García, F. and Sarriá, A. (2005). *Revisión de intervenciones con nuevas tecnologías en el control de las enfermedades crónicas [Review of the use of new technologies in the control of chronic diseases].* Madrid: AETS-ISCIII.

Goffman, E. (1989). *Estigma. La identidad deteriorada [Stigma. Notes on the Management of Spoiled Identity].* Buenos Aires: Amorrortu.

Haro, J.A. (2000). Cuidados profanos: una dimensión ambigua en la atención de la salud [Non professional care: an ambiguous dimension on healthcare]. I: Comelles, J.M. and Perdiguero, E. (eds.) *Medicina y Cultura. Estudios entre la Antropología y la Medicina.* Barcelona: Bellaterra. pp. 101-161.

Husserl, E. (1991). *La crisis de las ciencias europeas y la fenomenología transcendental. Una introducción a la filosofía fenomenológica [The crisis of the European sciences and transcendental phenomenology. An introduction to phenomenological philosophy].* Barcelona: Editorial Crítica.

Illich, I. (1975). *Némesis Médica. La expropiación de la salud [Medical Nemesis. The expropriation of health].* Barcelona: Barral Editores.

Kleinman, A. (1980). *Patients and Healers in the Context of Culture.* Berkeley: University of California Press.

Kleinman, A. (1987). *Social Contexts of Health, Illness and Patient Care*. Berkeley: California University Press.

Kleinman, J. (2000). El curso social del sufrimiento: esquizofrenia, epilepsia y otras enfermedades crónicas en la cultura china [The social course of suffering: schizophrenia, epilepsy and other chronic diseases in Chinese culture]. In: González, E. and Comelles, J.M. (comps.), *Psiquiatría Transcultural*. Madrid: Asociación Española de Neuropsiquiatría, 101-116.

Kleinman, A. and Benson, P. (2004). La vida moral de los que sufren enfermedad y el fracaso existencial de la medicina [The moral life of sufferers from an illness and the existential failure of medicine]. *Humanitas Monográfico* no. 2, pp. 17-26.

Law 16/2003, 28 May, of *Cohesion and Quality of the National Health System (NHS). [Cohesión y Calidad del Sistema Nacional de Salud, SNS]*, BOE Núm. 128, 29/05/03, pp. 20567-20588. Available at:
http://www.msc.es/organizacion/consejoInterterri/docs/LeyCohesionyCalidad.pdf
[accessed June 23 2009]

Law 39/2006. *Law for the promotion of personal autonomy and care for persons in a situation of dependency (Ley de promoción de la autonomía personal y atención a las personas en situación de dependencia)*. Ministry of Labor and Social Affairs. Ministerio de Trabajo y Asuntos Sociales (MTAS). BOE núm. 299, 15-12-2006. Available at: http://www.boe.es/aeboe/consultas/bases_datos/doc.php?coleccion=iberlex&id=2006/21990 and in
http://www.gencat.net/benestar/prodep/pdf/lleiestataldep.pdf [accessed June 23 2009]

López-Casasnovas, G. (2007). El papel del seguro sanitario y la medicina privada en los sistemas públicos de salud [The role of health insurance and private medicine in the public health system]. Humanitas. *Humanidades Médicas* (14), April, 11-25.

Mauss, M. (1971). Ensayo sobre los dones. Motivo y forma del cambio en las sociedades primitivas [(1923-1924) *Essai sur le don*. Forme et raison de l'échange dans les sociétés archaïques]. In: *Sociología y Antropología*, 2nd ed. Madrid: Tecnos, 153-263.

Menéndez, E. [1974] (1978). 'El modelo médico y la salud de los trabajadores.' [The medical model and the health of workers]. In: Basaglia, F. et al.: *La salud de los trabajadores. Aportes para una política de la salud*. [The health of workers: toward a politics of health]. México: Ed. Nueva Imagen, 11-51.

Menéndez, E. (1983). *Hacia una práctica médica alternativa. Hegemonía y autoatención (gestión) en salud [Towards an alternative form of medical practice. Hegemony and self-care]*. México: CIESAS, Cuadernos de la Casa Chata, 86.

Menéndez, E. (1992). Grupo doméstico y proceso salud/enfermedad/atención: del teoricismo al movimiento continuo [Domestic groups and health/sickness/care processes: from theoreticism to continuous motion]. *Cuadernos Médico Sociales*, 59: 3-18.

Menéndez, E. (2003). Modelos de atención de los padecimientos: de exclusiones teóricas y articulaciones prácticas [Models of care: theoretical exclusions and practical articulations]. *Ciencia & Saúde Colectiva*, 8(1):185-207.

Merleau-Ponty, M. [1945] (1993). *Fenomelogía de la percepción*. [Phenomenology of Perception.] Barcelona: Planeta.

Ministerial order for the creation of the program *'Living longer, living better': sociomedical care for elders with LTC diseases.* (*'Vida als anys' d'atenció sòcio-sanitària a la gent gran amb llarga malaltia*. ORDRE 29-05-1986, DOGC (694), 02-06-1986).

Nobel, G. (1991). Aspectos psicosociales del enfermo crónico [Psychcosocial aspects of chronic patients]. *Enfermería Psicosocial*; II: 239-241.

OMS (2006). *Estrategia Mundial sobre Régimen Alimentario, Actividad Física y Salud. Marco para el seguimiento y evaluación de la aplicación. [Global Strategy on Diet, Physical Activity and Health].* Ginebra, Organización Mundial de la Salud.

Parsons, T. (1999). *El sistema social [The social system].* Madrid: Alianza Editorial.

Perdiguero, E. (2004). El fenómeno del pluralismo asistencial: una realidad por investigar [The phenomenon of healthcare pluralism: a reality to be researched]. *Gaceta Sanitaria*; 18 (1): 140-145.

Singer, M. and Castro, A. (2004). Introduction*: Anthropology and health policy: a critical perspective*. I: Castro, A. and Singer, M. *Unhealthy Health Policy: A Critical Anthropological Examination.* Walnut Creek, CA: Altamira Press. pp. xi-xx.

WHO (2002). *Reducing risks, promoting healthy life.* Geneva, World Health Organization, Technical Report, 916.

WHO (2003). *Key Policy Issues in Long-Term Care.* Geneva, World Health Organization.

WHO (2004). *World Health Report 2004. Changing history.* Geneva, World Health Organization.

Rose-Anna Foley, Yannis Papadaniel, François Kaech, Ilario Rossi

## Chapter XIII.

# From curative to palliative care: Confronting the new medical realities in a hospitalised end of life

Hospitals are interesting settings to observe coexistence and interactions between various professional segments (Strauss, 1961, 1992), as well as changes and innovations within the medical field. While hospital caregivers share the same general aim of providing better care for the patient,[1] each unit has its own time-frame, organisation, priorities, rules, language, and its ways of coping with illness, recovery and death. Within these different paradigms, palliative care can be considered as a divergent or exceptional group, as its whole definition is based on its distinction from curative care. Its purpose is to relieve the person when death can be anticipated within a short time, and when there is little hope of a cure. Opposite to most medical services, palliative professionals are not specialised in a particular age group (new born, elderly, etc.), a specific part of the human body, or a specific illness.

Its specific focus on one crucial moment of life, when death is near, makes it quite difficult for the benefits of palliative care to be recognised, since incurable illness and death have always been part of a hospital's mission. Nevertheless, palliative care has developed by showing the need for a new way of considering and providing care for the dying. Its defenders reacted to the negative effects of the changes that have taken place in recent years, whereby 'dying' has been moved, as it were, from the home to the hospital. Nowadays, 80 % of a population in a Western urban context dies in hospitals.[2] This change happened without hospital caregivers being prepared for it, neither in regard to training, organisation, or care (Moulin, 2000). It led to what palliative care defenders considered to be a form of technical, inhuman care of the dying in hospital: situations were denounced in which hospitalised dying patients were considered as a burden and were either undergoing intensive, painful, curative treatments until death, or were abandoned by doctors incapable of communicating with them (Verspieren and Rapin, 1989). Alongside these protests from professionals, a strong critique emerged towards the medicalisation of death in our societies (Ariès, 1975; Elias, 1987; Aïach and Delanoë, 1998). In America, the important work of Glaser and Strauss (1965, 1968) documented the process of death occultation in hospitals by showing the caregivers' need to bring death under control through strong routines and technical work.

The aim of palliative care is to restore the dying person's dignity by offering a new vision of the patient's needs. The conception introduced by Cicely Saunders (1984) of 'total pain' shows the importance, in addition to the somatic medical response, of considering the spiritual, social and psychological suffering in a holistic vision of the person. In order to offer this, interdisciplinary teams are composed of various actors (doctors, nurses, chaplains, psychologists, social workers, art-therapists, volunteers) dedicated to the individual's specific needs. With this new representation of global care occurring at a time when biomedicine is going through an important crisis (Benoist, 1989), many professionals are eager to give a new meaning to their practice. In this sense, becoming a palliative care practitioner can correspond to the ideal of no longer focusing exclusively on the technical and biological aspects and considering each patient as an individual with specific needs, to which the practitioner should adapt.

The concept of palliative care can be considered as bio-psycho-social (Castra, 2003; Stiefel, 2007), which corresponds to one of the new models of care rapidly expanding in hospitals, cohabiting with the traditional bio-medical vision (Engel, 1977, 1997; Vanotti, 2006).[3] Thus, it can be assumed that this new sub-group fits in with the growing multiple medical realities adapting to plural social realities and no longer focusing on identical biological humans (Johannessen and Lazar, 2005). Through this paper we would like to discuss plurality within the hospital institution. Therefore, if we consider palliative care as a divergent medical segment, in which ways does it participate in medicine's renewal and represent an enlightener of interactions of intermedicality (Greene, 1998) within the medical field?

The institutionalisation of this new area of care is fragile. Palliative care has founded its identity on medicine's limitations (Castra, 2003) although wanting to fit into this field by becoming a recognised medical specialty. Within palliative organisations, a tension exists between generalising palliative care to caregivers from different backgrounds and, on the other hand, keeping it within separate units in order to preserve its original holistic model (Holden, 1980; Clark, 1994). Palliative care in specialised hospices was first developed in English-speaking countries within the operating margins of hospitals,[4] but currently, palliative care is more and more implanted in mobile teams (Mino, 2007) diffusing palliative philosophy and practice in hospital environments, at home or in elderly institutions.

While it has succeeded in developing an original model of care within independent hospices, palliative care is struggling to become integrated in hospitals, especially within the highly technical and scientific academic institutions (Castra, 2007, Legrand, 2007). What are the barriers to the promotion of this philosophy of care inside the medical institution? Is this poor recognition linked, as some palliative care defenders say, to an aversion towards death in our modern societies? Rather, are we facing a lack of interest in this a 'passive' discipline, which does not bring progress in fighting against illness and death? Or, should we consider palliative care as a young medical discipline which needs time to bring rather new and challenging values into the highly competitive and acute hospital setting?

In this chapter, we would first like to discuss the specificities of palliative work through the daily interactions between hospital caregivers and palliative professionals, as well as the frictions that emerge while attempting to integrate this new model of care in the hospital setting. Indeed, palliative care corresponds to a rather different medical reality because of its new conception of the illness trajectory,[5] translating core palliative values such as taking time to adapt to the patient's needs, while at the same time efficiently relieving the person from pain and end of life symptoms. Secondly, we will look at the institutional and political issues underlying these divergent realities, which influence recognition of palliative care within the medical field. Because the hospital institution requires strong adaptation, we will discuss the specific identity that mobile teams represent within palliative care and the risk that this new model of care might face if it adjusts more to the hospital as an institution, than to bringing change and renewal to it.

The reflections presented in this chapter are based on ethnographic fieldwork made from observations and interviews carried out in a Swiss teaching hospital. They are part of a larger nationally funded project[6] dedicated to the development of palliative care in a specific Swiss region within different institutions and associations, such as hospitals, elderly institutions, home care and volunteer associations.

## Fieldwork in a palliative hospital mobile team

In the teaching hospital observed, the palliative activity is represented by the mobile team unit of the palliative care service.[7] The particularities of the palliative mobile team include the fact that it doesn't have its own bed unit and therefore doesn't have direct responsibility for patients. Its professional activity depends on phone calls from 'first line'[8] professionals asking for help and advice in the care of incurable patients. The palliative care team, on demand, then goes into service, sees the patient and makes recommendations to the hospital caregivers.

Fieldwork consisted in following the in-hospital palliative care professionals during their daily activities, mainly while answering calls from various services such as internal medicine, surgery, radio-oncology, neurology, rheumatology, orthopedics or intensive care units. Fifty clinical consultations of patients, including recommendations to hospital professionals, were followed during an eighteen-month period.[9] The internal palliative activity consisted of daily reports, training, psychiatric supervisions, and developing research projects, and was of principal importance while the professionals were not on call. All activities were regularly attended; among these, seventy palliative internal daily transmission meetings. These observations were completed with face-to-face comprehensive interviews with the palliative care professionals,[10] as well as with caregivers from the internal medicine service, which is the palliative mobile team's major client.[11]

Concerning those patients who were being cared for by the palliative mobile team, most of them were at the very end of their life and in need of technical help, which cannot be offered in non-acute settings such as elderly institutions, regional hospitals, or at home. Because of the delicate situation they were in, informal discussions with patients and relatives were preferred to interviews during their hospital stay.[12] Interviews were also carried out, however, with relatives of those patients who had been seen by the palliative care mobile team and had died in the observed hospital at least a year prior to the interview.[13]

In the observed university hospital, 35,000 patients are admitted each year. Approximately 500 are seen by the palliative mobile team. Out of these patients, 200 pass away, representing 20 % of the institution's total deaths. If we consider exclusively palliative patients who died in that hospital in one year, only 38 % were looked after by the palliative care team.[14] This means few services are referring to the specialised team taking care of the dying in that hospital. These figures are surprising knowing that, in this specific region, the promotion of palliative care is a public health priority.[15] Hereafter, these results are questioned in the light of daily interactions and negotiations between the palliative professionals and the 'first line' caregivers referring to them.

ROSE-ANNA FOLEY, YANNIS PAPADANIEL, FRANÇOIS KAECH, ILARIO ROSSI

## Confronting incurable illness trajectories and work organisation

The emergence of palliative care has had an important impact on conceptions of the trajectories for incurable illness. With a strong critical point of view regarding the prolonging of life by medical means,[16] it has introduced the importance of a phase at the end of the incurable illness trajectory when healthcare professionals should cease trying to cure if there is little or no chance of healing the patient. In daily practice, this critical point of view is present in palliative care professionals' discourses when they denounce the use of tiring and painful invasive treatments (chemotherapy, radiotherapy, surgery, antibiotics, blood samples and injections) by doctors they encounter, who should rather focus on the patient's quality of life for the little time left. Palliative care professionals consider the doctors' wish to continue treatments to be a failure, and a way of denying the limitations of medicine, when there are poor chances of healing, and death is near. Palliative care's militant position (Castra, 2003, 2007) is to 'convince' hospital professionals to abandon this particular conception and renew their practice with palliative values and norms in end of life care. Among 'first line' professionals, many nurses and nurse aids already share the palliative vision because of their more humanistic and relational professional culture, and therefore represent important allies in suggesting to doctors that they refer to the palliative mobile team.[17]

However, even when 'first line' physicians are convinced about the new way of considering and acting on incurability, observations have shown there are difficulties in shifting from a curative perspective to a palliative one. The following discourse indicates it can be very demanding and difficult to apply the palliative attitude in the entirely diagnosis- focused and organised hospital institution. It requires that they no longer focus on ways to cure and instead switch to an approach based on the relief of patients' symptoms:

> I experienced two situations where I had missed the opportunity to call palliative care. I didn't see it go by. This happens to me when I have patients for a month or so. You follow them for a month, you invest a lot, then suddenly you feel that you can't hold on anymore and you lose a little focus. You are so concentrated on, 'Ok, let's treat the pneumonia, the kidney is not functioning', there are so many different specialists involved … And then suddenly I've had a situation where someone die in the same day and I had to do all the palliative care work during the same day. And then, I realised the patient didn't want to continue. In that situation I missed the boat. It's

difficult to feel how all of a sudden things change and the patient doesn't necessarily tell us. This is why it is highly important to have people who are involved in a new way with the patient (Tony, assistant doctor, internal medicine, translated from French).

An important moment in the newly formalised approach regarding incurable illness is when the palliative team is called. While palliative professionals wish to anticipate end of life in the best conditions by creating early partnerships that combine curative and palliative aspects of care, doctors tend to first ask for their intervention only when they themselves are out of resources and facing complex situations, most often the very end of life. The doctor's words presented here show how one can easily miss this phase of anticipation as well as the 'right moment' to exclude the curative approach in favour of the other. In line with a patient-centred model, the precise time to change course must also be defined by the patient's and relatives' wish to continue or stop curative treatments,[18] although, in the busy and acute setting of hospital units, there is often little time and space to scrutinise these needs. Thus, the palliative vision with its new consideration of the dying individual's needs, is challenging medical practice, hospital work and organisation rules.

### New controversial clinical knowledge

Another aspect of the palliative mission's focus on patients' demands and the relief of their suffering, is the important research on the specific use of medicines and treatments such as opioids (morphine and its derivates). These substances have been used in hospitals for a long time for acute pain, but palliative care has introduced them for chronic pain and incurability with a specific knowledge on dosage and rotation options. Fighting against end-of-life pain and successfully relieving patients represents the principal tool for proving palliative care's value within the medical institution (Castra, 2007).[19]

While the lack of palliative knowledge still causes deplorable situations of suffering and frequent medical error (often denounced during palliative daily internal reports), many hospital doctors recognise the utility of this new complex knowledge and appreciate being taught about it by the palliative professionals. On the other hand, there is some reluctance and disagreements about adapting treatments and following palliative care recommendations, due to strong side effects and social representations of the substances used. Among hospital professionals, palliative caregivers observe a general tendency of refusing to give high dosages of opioids or of considerably reducing the treatment as soon as the patient is feeling better, which generally has the negative effect of rapidly bringing pain back again.

The common belief that morphine can accelerate death or make the patient feel worse (dizzy, confused or addicted) is often expressed by non-palliative caregivers and mainly considered as linked to old, erroneous ideas that evidence-based researches have refuted. Nevertheless, most first-line caregivers speak of having encountered hospital caregivers afraid of administering these substances and of aggravating the situation: nurses and nurse aids spoke of doctors dreading the necessity of prescribing morphine and derivates. Assistant doctors identified head doctors' opposition towards these substances, whereas head doctors mainly pointed to nurses. Putting the blame on others could reveal that administering these substances to near-death patients remains problematic and inappropriate for some people, although it is now highly stigmatised to have such 'irrational' or 'false beliefs' within hospitals. However, according to most professionals, these ideas are diminishing more and more within hospitals, whereas the patients themselves and their families are considered to have the strongest reluctance towards morphine.[20]

Corresponding to a more recent practice, palliative sedation, which consists in putting a patient into controlled artificial sleep when pain symptoms cannot be relieved, is generating strong unambiguous reluctance. This action, often considered as slow euthanasia, raises controversial standpoints (Bilings and Block, 1996), although it is more and more recognised as an ethically justified palliative action in order to avoid intolerable suffering and agony.[21] Often called in situations of intense suffering and difficult agony, palliative professionals are considered by the client services as experts of palliative sedation. Nevertheless, two important barriers are identified: first, doctors and nurses are frequently unwilling to be part of the sleep induction process mostly due to the emotional cost of making someone who is close to death sleep, not knowing if the sedated person will wake up again. Secondly, some doctors go ahead with sedation at an earlier stage in the illness trajectory, without respecting the palliative expertise and vision of recourse to sedation, only and strictly, when there are no other therapeutic options available and death is near.

The reluctance towards palliative treatments and the misuses that result from this reluctance, reveal the embarrassment that incurability represents in the hospital setting. For doctors, who have been used to 'abandoning' dying patients, it seems that new dilemmas have emerged around the possibility of accelerating death or shortening agony, thanks to these powerful substances. They question the small margin between relieving and killing the patient with these substances, which are, the doctors believe, emblematic of medicine's uneasy intervention in treating a close to death patient.

## Palliative temporality and organisation as renewed care options

Because palliative care, with its specific way of considering the self and body, gives special attention to individual needs and the relational psycho-spiritual aspects of care, it implies a special time-frame which allows palliative professionals to spend more than an hour with a patient if needed, and visit only a few patients per day. Conversely, a 'first line' caregiver has many patients to look after, 24 hours a day, seven days a week, and it is rarely possible for them to spend much time with one patient.

The alternative palliative time-frame is often considered by hospital professionals as a way to improve care in an acute unit where priority must often be given to patients 'who can be saved'. Also, most professionals, be it nurses, nurse aids or doctors, agree that hospital is an inappropriate, impersonal and rather disturbing setting for accompanying dying patients and their relatives, and therefore they welcome possibilities that make up for these deficiencies. On the other hand, the different curative and palliative organisation can generate reactions from caregivers, who complain about the insufficient availability of the palliative mobile team who work only Mondays to Fridays during office hours (as they don't have a bed unit), leaving the hospital unit unstaffed at the weekends. Also, if palliative professionals can offer time to patients, their specific way of functioning can be particularly demanding for hospital doctors who have the least time to spend with patients:

> The first day, when we make an appointment with the palliative care team, we know it will take time. We calculate one or two hours. The [palliative] nurse will sometimes come twice a day to see the patient, the assistant [doctors] sometimes have an hour to talk about religious things for example. If I start talking about that, it's Pandora's box. I can't stop the patient. We just don't have the structure for it. Because officially we have nine minutes per patient for the entire visit, talk to the nurse, everything. For all the rest, we count on extra hours. It is limited. We don't feel economic restrictions, but time is the main factor. We will do something if we have time to do it, otherwise too bad (Tony, Assistant doctor, Internal Medicine, translated from French).

Beyond the confrontation with a very rigid and constraining time-frame based on efficiency and acute care, the specific consultant organisation seems to disturb the classical model of biomedical doctor/patient relationship causing role overlapping and difficulties in defining respective competence fields. When a new doctor spending time with the patient arrives, there is a risk of losing some aspects of the relationship initially created with the patient. Also, a sense of failing to do one's duty in properly looking after a patient until death can be felt when it is necessary to refer to a consultant team. It is interesting that a type of 'dispossession' is also present in the palliative discourses, as some doctors find it frustrating to have to accept the role of adviser and not be in charge of the whole clinical situation themselves.

The process of having two teams working for the same patient goes against values of doctors' deontology, such as responsibility and autonomy. For instance, some hospital nurses speak of doctors' difficulties in asking for a palliative expert's advice, as this may imply an incapacity to look after a patient in an autonomous way. Collaboration and networking are not specific to the interactions between the palliative and curative sectors. It can be considered as a growing mode of interaction, gaining more and more importance in the biomedical field, be it between general practitioners and specialists, psychiatrists and other paramedical professions (social workers, physiotherapists), or simply between doctors, nurses and nurse aids (Rossi, 2002). Nevertheless, palliative care is introducing new values such as mutual help, considering the physician's emotional experience while taking care of incurable and dying patients. Indicating that this change is welcome, although challenging traditional professional habits, one doctor said it was rather surprising and amusing that palliative physicians cared for their inner experience of caring for dying patients, while complaining that doctors – in comparison with nurses, who tend to stand by each other – are too often left alone to deal with their emotions.

Palliative care professionals are developing important expertise in communication around end-of-life experience, death and grief. They have at their disposal many internal spaces for reflection and discussion about their professional activity and human experience of taking care of dying patients (such as psychiatric supervisions, reflective work groups, informal discussions with palliative colleagues including a psychologist and a chaplain). Also, they are often identified by 'first line' colleagues as powerful mediators when patients and families have divergent ways of experiencing incurability, or if hospital professionals disagree among themselves about the incurable illness trajectory and possible medical interventions. Illustrating this, one assistant doctor mentioned that he immediately called the palliative team when a colleague who was also involved in an end-of-life situation was 'less sensitive' to the palliative approach. In the same way, when a patient is showing obvious signs of death denial, or if the person is anxious about the moment of death, the palliative caregivers are called, as it is perceived that they have the proper experience and training to talk about death.

So, even if there is tension concerning the amount of time the 'palliative' and the 'curative' personnel can spend with a patient, and the multiplication of actors around the same patient might not match the classical doctor-patient relationship, expertise in communication and the availability of time for the patient seem to be of importance for doctors choosing to use the services of the palliative mobile team. The above can be considered visible aspects of change and renewal brought about by palliative care's intervention in hospital services for incurability and death. The ideal of the 'good death' seems to have shifted from *the absence of words*, in order to control death and protect one from its emotional consequences (Glaser and Strauss, 1965, 1968; Herzlich, 1976), to the importance of *talking about the experience* of dying and grief, in order to deal with its consequences in the most suitable way.

## Is there space in the hospital institution for new medical reality, and at what cost?

If palliative care offers an opportunity for change and renewal in hospitals, its activity is strongly dependant on the curative services' making daily requests for their help. Should first-line caregivers not be satisfied with the palliative recommendations, they can simply decline to adopt the treatments, or, if disagreements are too strong, they will not use the services of the palliative mobile team again. In this teaching hospital, there is neither a clear direction, nor official procedure regarding palliative care referrals. It is up to each service to deal with and take decisions about the dying patients they admit. For example, the head doctor of a service may only first ask his staff to call the palliative care mobile team when facing complex situations with dying patients. Another could refer to the palliative care team as soon as incurability is diagnosed, whereas a third unit will develop its own palliative care vision without using the services of the palliative mobile team.

Underlying these aspects, there are political and economic issues regarding territoriality and recognition mechanisms within the hospital institution. The arrival of a new specialty on the hospital scene generates power struggles for recognition and institutional status (Strauss, 1961, 1992). The creation of a new department changes the conditions of exercising medicine and the production of medical knowledge (Pinell, 2005). It is equal to a new distribution of patients within the different wards. The service that has the most beds is also the one that has the most power in the institution: the number of patients admitted in a unit determines the number of doctors employed and therefore defines its importance and acknowledgment within the institution. The fact that the palliative care service in this hospital does not have a bed unit is in itself a factor revealing its minor influence in the institution.[22]

More generally, Strauss (1961, 1992) shows that there are always conflicts or at least differences of interests within the medical profession. These lead to coalitions and cleavages in opposition to other specialties or medical segments. The biomedical field is undergoing constant change and, as boundaries become diffuse and generations overlap, new groupings may emerge (Strauss, 1961: 332). Early in its development, a new segment often proclaims its unique mission and can tend to have a rather evangelistic position, whereas an old segment will have a more defensive position as it is forced to reaffirm some aspects of its identity. Furthermore, when a specialty arises, it often exploits a new method or technique, or relationship to the patient (Strauss, 1961: 329). Palliative care professionals, while dealing with the patient's inner experience of end of life (Castra, 2007), use the relationship to patients as a complex therapeutic tool, which gives them the status of experts in this field.

If palliative care has the main distinctive features of a new medical specialty, it cannot easily be assumed that one day it will become a fully-fledged segment of medicine because of its fundamental divergent palliative philosophy. In the past, not much was done by doctors for incurable patients. Nurses were mainly in charge of them as they did not raise any interesting medical problem (Pinell, 2005). Nowadays, there seems to be greater attention paid to patients with severe illness, but are we not facing the same old problem with biomedicine remaining resolutely built on values of healing and progress (Strauss et al., 1997)? Whereas most new specialties emerge with new technologies, which hope to fight diseases more effectively, palliative care does not bring innovative ways to eradicate illness and death. Its new clinical knowledge only has the aim to relieve suffering and it cannot fight against the progression of the disease. If we add to this the fact that palliative care that is based on individual needs 'costs' a lot of time, it appears that it is inadequate when compared with the hospital's fast and acute activity.

According to Mino et al. (2008), this medicine of incurability will not survive without the help of politicians and administrators creating institutional projects in training and quality care processes. Nevertheless, there could be some hope as this new model of care is gaining more and more popularity within lay opinion. According to this author, the creation of palliative mobile teams within hospitals is already a sign of this change. As well known, values such as quality of life and respect for the patient are strong public demands that are addressed to medicine especially since the appearance of cancer.

In Switzerland, where assisted suicide is tolerated, associations such as Exit are also gaining favourable public opinion and have recently been allowed in some university hospitals. However, palliative care appears as a more socially acceptable practice and has become a national Public Health priority. Also, institutionalisation outside the university hospital in the specific region[23] observed, including one palliative care hospice, four external mobile teams, two palliative care bed units within regional hospitals, and several volunteer associations, shows that this particular medical reality is gaining more and more importance.[24]

In the hospital, pressures linked to institutional recognition and collaboration with curative services are of major importance. Palliative care professionals have to adapt to the biomedical structure's rules in order to gain recognition. Communication and diplomacy skills are of prime importance in order to perpetuate the precious collaboration with hospital services (Legrand, 2007). The more the palliative professionals are called, the more their activity will develop and their influence will grow in the institution. Isn't there a risk, however, that these aspects may become more primordial than the humanistic patient-centred vision of care? What is the place for the hospitalised dying patient's needs when, as shown, caregivers are preoccupied with issues to do with collaboration, implementing new models of care and integration in the hospital structure? The fact that several palliative professionals expressed their frustration with not being able to focus entirely on the patient, reveals the tension between creating a meaningful humanistic doctor/patient relationship and, on the other hand, the need to concentrate on collaboration, the diffusion of palliative care philosophy, and institutional issues.

However, among the observed palliative mobile team, some professionals claim their specific consultant role (Teike-Lüthi and Gallant, 2007) as clinical expertise and support to hospital professionals, rather than ongoing direct care to incurable patients. More generally, palliative mobile teams, whether they evolve in hospitals, at home or in elderly institutions have a common pedagogical mission to bring new clinical and relational tools, reflexivity and support to 'first line' professionals. This means that diplomacy precautions and communication skills are part of the palliative mobile teams' specific identity and role in generalising palliative care. Compared to existing independent palliative care structures, a great heterogeneity of practices can be noticed. For example, specialised palliative hospices give more importance to global care. There are several spiritual and religious activities and a place is given to complementary and alternative medicines (Gadri, 2002; Foley, 2006). In the academic hospital, the trend is to stick to the more pragmatic aspects of care. Within the observed palliative mobile team, there are evident signs of a distinction process from the more orthodox palliative care vision as it was developed in hospices. For instance, hospital palliative professionals reject the most esoteric aspects of care while claiming a more serious and scientific palliative approach. If the several quantitative and more recently qualitative research projects developed in this service are the reflection of adaptation strategies to fit into the hospital, it also corresponds to the wish of developing a reflexive and professional culture having its place in the hegemonic hospital setting, and no longer considered only as a compassionate and rather unscientific practice.

Regarding the above, many palliative defenders perceive the risk that, while adapting to the hospital institution, palliative care might have to abandon its bio-psycho-social model in favour of a more biomedical focus on somatic treatments. Thus, making palliative care more scientific introduces the risk of reinforcing the biomedical paradigm traditionally separating *soma* from *psyche*, rather than introducing the human being in its wholeness. It would also question the need for interdisciplinary teams including chaplains, social workers and volunteers within hospitals. At some point, generalising palliative care could result in reducing this new model to basic clinical knowledge and tools that all caregivers can use without having to refer to palliative experts anymore. The threat of palliative care's disappearance is all the more palpable in hospitals where mobile teams are put to the test by the hegemonic biomedical institution and undergo important pressure while trying to become a recognised medical specialty. Palliative work and its intervention on incurable patients are confronting the hospital's organisational rules and raise important dilemmas for the caregivers facing 'condemned' patients. Nevertheless, it offers long temporality to patients, new communication skills to professionals, and opportunities to have a reflective look at their way of interacting with patients and going through the highly emotional care of the dying, which shows nuances and renewal opportunities between these confrontational medical realities.

# Notes

1   We must not forget, however, that hospitals are not representative of one global biomedical model. They can take different forms depending on the culture, and reflecting and reinforcing the core values and beliefs of a culture (Van der Geest and Finkler, 2004).

2   Although nowadays there is an important promotion of dying at home and a strong wish from patients to be cared for at home (Favrot-Laurens 1996), many deaths still take place in hospital due to the need for hospital techniques at the very end of life, and also because of the burden for families who have to look after a dying parent at home.

3   Following what Engel developed in his work (1977, 1997), the importance of considering bio-psycho-social aspects in care was confirmed by the World Health Organisation in 1998 in its *Framework for Professional and Administrative Development of General Practice / Médecine de famille en Europe*, WHO Europe, Copenhagen. According to Vanotti (2006), nowadays, three models cohabitate in hospital: the biomedical, the bio-psycho-social and the systemic model corresponding to the psychiatric influence.

4   The first palliative care hospice in Great Britain created in 1967 by C. Saunders, the St-Christopher's Hospice, rapidly became a worldwide known model in terms of palliative care and initiated what is since considered as the Hospice Movement.

5   The term *trajectory* is used according to Strauss's definition to refer to the *organisation of work* done during the illness in contrast with the common sense and professional term of *course of illness* (Strauss et al., 1997).

6   National funded project 100013-112411/1: 'Life medicalisation and death management: palliative care development as a social and cultural issue', directed by Prof. I. Rossi in collaboration with F. Kaech and Y. Papadaniel.

7   The palliative care service, which was created in 1996, is composed of an internal mobile team working within the hospital and an external mobile team visiting patients at home and within elderly institutions. Our observations are based on the internal mobile team's activity. This team is composed of a professor doctor, one head doctor, two clinician head doctors, two assistant doctors, one head nurse, one clinician nurse, two nurses, a psychologist, a chaplain and a social worker.

8   This indigenous term will be used between brackets to distinguish the palliative professionals from the hospital caregivers, who have direct responsibility for patients and are therefore referred to as 'first line' professionals.

9   Having the choice of either joining staff, patients or visitors while doing ethnographic research in the hospital (Van der Geest and Finkler, 2004), we chose to be introduced as a research team in anthropology, collaborating on a nationally funded project. The hospital's ethics committee, as well as the palliative professionals, decided we should hand the patient an informed consent for signing before entering his room. Before interviewing each hospital professional, we also had to follow the procedure of informed consent. Regarding the constraints and consequences of this procedure, see Rossi et al., 2007, 2008. Rose-Anna Foley was in charge of ethnographic fieldwork within the hospital. It is also the subject of her doctorate thesis, which focuses on the representations and uses of palliative medicines as analysers of incurable illness' experience and palliative practice within hospital. After more than a year following the palliative mobile team, she started collaborating as a researcher within

the palliative service. About the stakes and implications of this activity, while keeping the anthropologist's critical view see Canevascini and Foley 2009.

10 Nine interviews were carried out with members of the in-hospital palliative care mobile team and included the head doctor, a clinician head doctor, an assistant doctor, the head nurse, the clinician nurse, one of the nurses, the psychologist, the chaplain and the social worker.

11 Twelve professionals (four clinician head doctors, two assistant doctors, one head nurse, three nurses, and two nurse aids) from the Internal Medicine unit were interviewed.

12 Patients were sometimes too fragile and suffering so much pain that they could not hold a pen and sign the informed consent presented to them. Many of them were already unconscious when the palliative team was asked to take part. In some cases however, the patients' suffering was controlled and some could go back home, while regularly consulting the palliative professionals during ambulatory visits. In those cases, we were able to have more in-depth discussions with patients and relatives after the palliative visit.

13 This procedure allows next of kin to have time to go through the first and most intense phases of mourning before being asked to participate in an interview. Among respondents who agreed to be interviewed, the majority said they had only recently been able to talk about their deceased loved one without too much emotion. Up to now, seven of approximately twenty interviews have been carried out with family members of deceased patients.

14 These figures are based on an ongoing study in collaboration with the palliative service of the observed hospital (Beauverd *et al.*, 2008). In this research, the difficulty to find a precise definition of palliative patients was raised. The figure presented here corresponds to a minimal definition of palliative care according to ten typical palliative diagnoses. About this definition, see McNamara *et al.*, 2006.

15 Regarding palliative care in the specific region observed, see: *Programme cantonal de développement des soins palliatifs* (2004).

16 Euthanasia movements, appearing at the same time as palliative care, shared the same point of view with the difference that palliative philosophy promoted quality of life while preserving it, which wasn't the case of euthanasia movements (La Marne, 1999).

17 In this university hospital, calls to the palliative team must be made by a doctor. Nurses are entitled to call palliative nurses for advice but cannot ask the palliative team to enter a situation without having the doctor's approval.

18 Patients and relatives can play an active part in calling the palliative mobile team or refusing to be seen by these end-of-life care specialists. Patients and relatives might disagree among themselves about stopping curative treatments, thus allowing oneself or a relative to die, etc. For the purpose of this article, we focus more on the professionals' perspective in order to analyse their point of views and actions as representative of the medical realities to which they belong.

19 Although palliative care has introduced pain as a global notion considering individual somatic, psychological, social and spiritual suffering, in hospital practice, however, suffering is most frequently reduced to its somatic relief by hospital professionals asking for palliative expertise. Nevertheless, palliative professionals set great emphasis on communication skills' allowing them to develop empathic caring. The team's psychologist and chaplain are also regularly included in the palliative intervention.

20 Among patients, opioids (especially morphine) are often considered as poisons rather than therapeutics. Many complain of strong side effects, hallucinations, or a feeling of being drugged. According to palliative and curative caregivers, some patients, especially among the elderly, express the *need* to feel some pain while suffering from incurable illness. This is often problematic for caregivers who try to convince the patient to take the treatment. In our national-funded project and the doctorate thesis on palliative care in hospitals (R.-A. Foley), special attention and focus is given to the role of palliative medicines in understanding what people suffering from severe and incurable illness go through.

21 Palliative sedation is often considered by palliative professionals as a way to prevent from euthanasia and assisted suicide when repeated death wishes are expressed by patients. Regarding assisted suicide, which is tolerated in Switzerland, the palliative care organisations take a strong position against it, affirming the natural course of life and the importance of accompanying people towards death even when they wish their life shortened.

22 Another sign of institutionalisation is the existence of a specialised Chair symbolising the recognition of the speciality by the academic authorities (Pinell, 2005). This generally, then, allows the specialty to be represented in the training centres, which is very important for recruiting and socialising young doctors (Strauss, 1961). The ultimate step in establishing power is the representation of the specialty members in ethics committees, certification procedures and professional associations (Strauss, 1961). This process is barely beginning for the palliative team observed, which recently opened the first Chair of palliative care in Switzerland. At the moment, it is only starting to be part of the training process of the Faculty of Medicine.

23 The Canton of Vaud (VD) is part of the French part of Switzerland. It has more than 650,000 inhabitants.

24 Also, international comparative studies realised by Clark *et al.* show that palliative care, although still widely insufficient, has rapidly developed since the 1960s and is becoming more recognised by policy-makers around the world (Clark, 2007; Wright et al., 2008).

## Bibliography

Aïach, P. and Delanoë D. (1998). *l'ère de la médicalisation, Ecce homo sanitas.* Paris: éd. Economica.

Ariès, P. (1975). *Essais sur l'histoire de la mort en Occident, du Moyen Age à nos jours.* Paris: Seuil.

Beauverd M., Foley R.-A., Rossi I. and Pereira J. (2008). Utilisation of palliative care consult service in a Swiss hospital: a caution note on determining the palliative population, presented at the Annual Day of consensus of the Swiss Society for Palliative Medicine and Care (Palliative.ch), Bienne, Switzerland, December 2008.

Benoist, J., (1989). *Introduction à la dimension culturelle de la maladie: quelques approches.* Toulouse: AMADES.

Billings, J.A. and Block, S.D. (1996). Slow euthanasia. *Journal of Palliative Care*, 12, (4): 21-30.

Canevascini, M. and Foley, R.-A. (2009). L'anthropologie face aux demandes du terrain: deux exemples d'implication dans le milieu médical, *Altérités*, in press.

Castra, M. (2003). *Bien mourir: Sociologie des Soins Palliatifs*, Paris: PUF.

Castra, M. (2007). Les équipes mobiles de soins palliatifs, entre expertise et "entreprise morale". *Revue Sociologie Santé*, 27: 52-66.

Clark, D. (2007). From margins to centre: a review of the history of palliative care in cancer, *Lancet Oncology*, 8: 430-438.

Clark, D. (1994). At the crossroads: which direction for the hospices? *Palliative Medicine*, 8, (1): 1-3.

Elias, N. (1987). *La solitude des mourants*. Paris: Christian Bourgeois.

Engel, G.L. (1977). The need for a new medical model: a challenge for biomedicine, *Science*, 196, 4286: 129-36.

Engel, G.L. (1997). From biomedical to biopsychosocial, being scientific in the human domain. *Psychosomatics*, 36, 6: 521-528.

Favrot-Laurens, G. (1996). Soins familiaux ou soins professionnels? La construction des catégories dans la prise en charge des personnes âgées dépendantes. In: Kaufmann, J.-C., *Faire ou faire-faire? Famille et services*. Rennes: Presses Universitaires de Rennes: 231- 252.

Foley, R.-A. (2006). L'accompagnement spirituel: entre dispositif de prise en charge et absence de discours, INFO*Kara*, *Revue internationale francophone de soins palliatifs*, 21, (3): 109-113.

Gadri, A. (2002). *Donner naissance à la mort*, Villeneuve, Mont-sur-Lausanne: Ouverture.

Glaser, B. and Strauss A. (1965). *Awareness of Dying*. Chicago: Aldine.

Glaser, B. and Strauss A. (1968). *Time for Dying*. Chicago: Aldine.

Greene, S. (1998). The Shaman's Needle: Development, Shamanic Agency, and Intermedicality in the Aguaruna Lands, Peru. *American Ethnologist*, vol. 25, (4): 634-658.

Herzlich, C. (1976). Le travail de la mort, *Annales. Economies, Sociétés, Civilisations*, 31, (1): 197-217.

Holden, C. (1980). The Hospice Movement and Its Implications, *The ANNALS of the American Academy of Political and Social Science*, 447: 59-63.

Johannessen, H. and Lazar I. (eds.), (2005). *Multiple medical realities, patients and healers in biomedical, alternative and traditional medicine*. New-York, Oxford: Berghahn Books.

La Marne, P. (1999). *Ethiques de la fin de vie, acharnement thérapeutique, euthanasie, soins palliatifs*. Paris: Ellipses.

Legrand, E. (2007). Des résistances à l'ingérence des Equipes Mobiles de Soins Palliatifs dans les services hospitaliers. *Sociologie Santé*, 26: 337-349.

McNamara, B., Rosenwax, L., D'arcy, J. and Holman, C. (2006). A method for defining and estimating the palliative care population. *Journal of Pain and Symptom Management*, 32, 1: 5-12.

Mino, J.-C., Frattini M.-O. and Fournier E. (2008). Pour une médecine de l'incurable. *Sociétés*, 408, (6): 753-764.

Mino, J.-C. (2007). Entre urgence et accompagnement, les équipes mobiles de soins palliatifs. *Sciences sociales et Santé*, 25, (1): 63-92.

Moulin, P. (2000). Les soins palliatifs en France: un mouvement paradoxal de médicalisation du mourir contemporain. *Cahiers Internationaux de Sociologie*, CVIII: 125-159.

Pinell, P. (2005). Champ médical et processus de spécialisation. *Actes de la recherche en sciences sociales*, 156-157: 4-36.

*Programme cantonal de développement des soins palliatifs, information à l'intention des professionnels de la santé.* Santé Publique, Etat de Vaud, 2004 (2nd ed.), 16 p.

Rossi, I. (2002). Réseaux de soins, réseaux de santé. Culture prométhéenne ou liberté de l'impuissance. *Tsantsa, revue de la Société Suisse d'Ethnologie*, 7: 12-21.

Rossi, I., Papadaniel Y., Kaech F. and Foley, R.-A. (2007). Les figures multiples de l'éthique: La mort entre médecine et société. *Tsantsa, revue de la Société Suisse d'Ethnologie*, 12: 136-141.

Rossi, I., Kaech, F., Foley, R.-A. and Papadaniel, Y. (2008). L'éthique à l'épreuve d'une enquête anthropologique en milieu palliatif: de l'insertion à la restitution, *Ethnographiques.org*, [on line], http://www.ethnographiques.org/2008/Rossi,et-al.html

Saunders, C. (1984). *Living with dying: the management of terminal disease*, London, New-York, Oxford: University Press.

Stiefel, F. (2007). *Soins palliatifs: une pratique aux confins de la médecine.* Paris: L'Harmattan.

Strauss, A. (1961). Professions in Process. *The American Journal of Sociology*, 66, (4): 325-334.

Strauss, A. (1992). *La trame de la négociation. Sociologie qualitative et interactionnisme.* Paris: L'Harmattan.

Strauss, A., Fagerhaugh, S., Suczek, B. and Wiener, C. (1997). *Social organisation of medical work.* New Jersey: Transaction Publishers.

Teike-Lüthi F. and Gallant, S. (2007). A consulting partnership, a relationship to be defined. *Recherche en Soins Infirmiers*, 90: 67-74.

Van der Geest, S. and Finkler, K. (2004). Hospital ethnography: introduction. *Social Science and Medicine*, 59: 1995-2001.

Vanotti M. (2006). *Le métier de médecin.* Genève: Médecine et hygiène.

Verspieren P. and Rapin C.-H. (eds), (1989). *Fin de vie, Nouvelles perspectives pour les soins palliatifs.* Lausanne: éd. Payot.

Wright, M., Wood, J., Lynch, T. and Clark, D. (2008). Mapping levels of palliative care development: a global view. *Journal of Pain and Symptom Management*, 35, (5): 469-485.

Els van Dongen

Chapter XIV.

# Cancer and integrity. Dealing with fragile realities

*Being a patient is not so difficult*
*It is more difficult to save your soul*

## Introduction

Cancer is known by its fragmentation, uncertainty and not-knowing. In the lives of cancer sufferers and their families and friends the threat of fragmentation becomes a fundamental experience, one that continuously assaults a person's 'illusion of wholeness'. Sometimes people are seriously ill; then again they feel healthy. Doctors and patients never know if the cancer has disappeared after treatment or whether it will return and how. Though death awaits us all, and we do not know when it will come, cancer patients consciously live under the shadow of finality. Life can no longer be taken for granted.

In times of cancer, the integrity of the body and the person is deeply affected; the world seems destroyed. Realities are not durable but fragile, confronting and conflicting. How do people deal with this complexity and variations and how, in the face of it, do they create a certain coherence in their lives?

There is much more at stake than a disease that takes a great deal of the world's medical efforts in research, care and treatment. Fragmentation, uncertainty and multiple realities unmake the world. The patient and her family will have to remake their world 'in addition' to the struggle of surviving the disease.

Grappling with cancer not only involves dealing with various physiological explanations and actions and differing, sometimes conflicting, medical realities. It also involves diverse expectations of those involved, a range of moral and practical issues (see for example Hunt, 1998), changing relationships, loss, deep emotions such as hopes and fears, stigma and loneliness.

The contradictory public discourse on 'the leprosy of modern times' (Sontag, 1978), the heroic metaphors of survivors, or fighting spirits or victors (cf. Weiss, 1997), just to name a few, often put an extra burden on people's shoulders. 'Doing cancer' is a delicate process for all who are involved. How can we deal with it? What is 'really at stake', to speak in Kleinman's words?

In anthropology, there is a variety of literature on the 'pragmatics' of dealing with illness, especially on the ways people interpret what happens and what has to be done. People are not passive sufferers; they are not paralysed. They are actively involved in choices of treatment, and try to control their situation. I will describe some of these actions. However, to me this seems only the beginning of our study. To be a patient is sometimes less difficult than to save your soul. In suffering we have to face how hard we have to struggle to maintain our integrity (cf. Kleinman, 2006) and to remain a person, i.e. to be a soul (cf. Hacking, 1995). We have to deal with uncertainty (Whyte, 1997) and face the inadequacy of our attempts to make a good life for ourselves and others. In what follows, I dwell on these difficult matters and reflect on my work as an anthropologist. At moments of 'intense pressure' and fragile realities, which can suddenly change, we can lose our social and personal integrity. Mostly, it does not happen. What do people do to prevent losing this integrity?

## Multiple medical realities – threats to integrity: some auto-ethnography

Life-threatening diseases, such as cancer, mobilise entire networks of family members, friends, and health professionals who try to make sense of what is happening and what has to be done. One of the first questions a patient and the family ask the doctor after having heard the final diagnosis is: 'What can be done?' This question comes even before 'making sense' of the illness. In our first encounter with the oncologist, he remarked: 'We cannot speculate about the causes of your disease but we can better ask: "what can be done"?'

We, my husband and I, wait in front of the surgeon's office. We wait for two hours looking at other patients who enter and leave and we watch the cartoons for children on the small television screen above our heads. A nurse comes now and then and tells us that we will have to wait a little longer... She apologizes. We are in the regional hospital which is familiar to us because the pace and tone of life of our small community also resonates within the walls of the hospital and because we have been here to play music in the Sunday services for patients. I have never been there as a patient. We greet people we know. This world is familiar and unknown at the same time.

We already know what kind of news the surgeon will bring because we had a long talk with our family doctor, who had received the results of the tests and he told us that I had colon cancer with a substantial metastasis in the liver. My prospects are bad. I received my status as an incurable cancer patient in my living room on a sunny afternoon.

The diagnosis took almost two months of visits to the hospital for examinations. I met radiologists, laboratory personnel and nurses, each having their own approach to the patient and his disease. One moment I cry in the arms of a nurse-assistant in the radiology department; another moment I lie totally dependent on a bed for a liver biopsy. One moment I am a human being with emotions and fears; the next moment my body is an object, of which certain interior parts are made visible on a screen that the doctor and I look at with great interest – but in different ways. My disease changes with every meeting. My pain increases.

The journey to the diagnosis was marked with x-rays, endoscopy, CT scans, biopsies and blood tests, each making visible – and thus making real – what is going on, but each time it was slightly different. For the first internist, specialised in diseases such as Crohn, it was a 'process' because she did not find cancer cells in the colon biopsy. For the radiologist, the disease was in my liver. To the surgeon it was my colon that mattered and required urgent action. In the meantime, we had to deal with other realities outside the hospital. Our children, family and friends gradually came to know that I had this disease, which is so often characterised by its fatal outcome.

Finally, the nurse who had apologised so much lets us enter into a small, sober room with a chair, a bed and a computer. My husband and I sit on the bed leaving the chair for the surgeon. After a while the surgeon enters. We shake hands. He starts the images of the CT scan: 'Well eh, I am sorry. I don't have good news; it doesn't look so good.' He runs the images at high speed and I see the slices of the interior of my body: 'Don't you see?' he asks, pro forma. No. I do not. It doesn't make sense to me. 'This is not typical of colon cancer', he adds. I: 'Oh? So, it isn't colon cancer? They haven't found cancer cells in the biopsies of the tissue, you know.' It is my hope that speaks. 'That's true, it made us unsure, but this is more serious', he said, showing slices of my liver. 'There is a major metastasis, the biopsy showed us that it is colon cancer.' Suddenly, I do not want to know the ins and outs of the slices. I do not care about the doctor's technical explanations. I get a flash of finality and of the depth of grief of my family and friends. All I can think of is 'not now, not me, not us...' I want to know what can be done and start to ask questions as well as I can. My husband also has his own questions. Everything seems unreal to me. 'We cannot cure you. We can try to control the cancer. Perhaps you will have some years left. I will have to operate on the colon as soon as possible, before I go on holiday... The liver cannot be operated, I know because I have done several such operations in the university hospital. In the meantime, you will have to make an appointment with the oncologist.' Holiday? Operation? A couple of years in the best scenario? University hospital? The doctor makes his plan for the surgery. I feel my husband tremble. We shake hands with the doctor again and leave... We sit in front of the secretary's desk to make the appointment for pre-op examinations and wait again, totally confused and silent. She phones a colleague and tells the story of her holidays and pregnancy. It is bizarre but we do not say a word; we have our own misery, which now slowly starts to unmake our common day-to-day world.

Within a few weeks, I was on the list for surgery. In that time, we also visited the oncologist. His manner was different from that of the surgeon. During these conversations I got the impression that he wanted to know what kind of a person I was. He asked what kind of work I did and we talked about medical anthropology. He asked me to bring something to read about this subject the next time, which I did (I would rethink my work and that of my colleagues many times during the episodes of my illness, wondering if the claims medical anthropology makes were just. He discussed the different options I had and stressed the 'free choice' I had. I was also offered participation in a clinical trial. The latter gave rise to wrenching uncertainty. Should I participate? I felt morally obliged to give my small contribution, but I felt desperate after I read the side-effects of the chemo. I could not decide. The oncologist made the final decision not to participate, saying 'You have done enough...' But what did I do?

I had surgery on the colon. The operation went well and I received a permanent marker on my body that would remind me that I belonged to 'the village of the sick' (Stoller, 2004). Perhaps it is an odd thing to write, but I remember this time in the hospital as a good time. The nurses tried to do everything to preserve my integrity, my limitations were respected and accommodated: they tried to give more than just physical care. Whenever they had some time, they came into my room for a talk or just to sit; they allowed my husband to come early in the morning to help me with showering and the new ritual I had to learn. Sometimes my room resembled a 'normal' living room. Of course, I cried a lot, I had my fears and – in particular – I worried about my family, seeing them sad, tired and uncertain. I could not bear to have friends at my hospital bed, but my refusal caused me moral problems too. I lived in two worlds: that of the sick and that of the healthy.

In the regional hospital as well as in the cancer clinic visits, the myriad of examinations, controls, MRI-scans, etc. were never a lonely enterprise. They were social events. There would be at least one family member or friend accompanying the patient, sometimes more. The examination rooms and offices of doctors always seemed to have at least two extra chairs. The crowded waiting spaces made me fear that waiting times could be long, but with every visit at least two persons went into the doctor's room.

Two weeks after the diagnosis we visited the oncologist again. We told him that we would 'go for the Lance Armstrong-variant',[1] which probably would bring strength and endurance. We wanted to have the best possible treatment. The oncologist frowned but scheduled me for several chemotherapies. Then we received an unexpected phone call from the surgeon of the cancer clinic in Rotterdam. It turned out that the surgeon of the regional hospital had sent the CD with the scan pictures to this clinic. It seemed he was not as confident as he pretended to be. This phone call turned our world upside-down again. The surgeon told us that he could operate my liver if the chemo-therapy worked well. I received two different kinds of chemo-therapy, stumbled through the days of nausea, weakness, tiredness, felt social isolation and strong emotions of uneasiness.

But they worked, and the ensuing liver operation went well. Within six days I was at home and tried to take my daily walks again. When we met the surgeon for a control visit, he said: 'We took half of your liver. Most of the tissue was necrosis with just a few cancer cells. We also took you gall bladder. The glands were clean. The part we took from the liver did not function anymore. So… go ahead and drink your wine in a couple of weeks.' This we did! My brother came from France with a bottle of champagne. We had to learn to be healthy again.

However, after a couple of weeks I began to suffer from terrible pains. Again I had examinations: a CT-scan to see if there was a new tumour – there was – radiation and chemo therapy to reduce the size of the tumour, a MRI-scan to precisely locate the tumour and another operation. I discovered that excruciating pain unmakes the social and moral world (cf. Scarry, 1985). It made me indifferent to what happened outside and even inside myself.

It was a difficult time for many people in my network, in particular for my children and husband.

We were in and out of the cancer clinic for weeks, every day during radiation treatment, and I started to feel better, the pain disappeared. 'You will have to trust yourself', the surgeon told me when he explained the operation to us, answering my remark that I would have to trust him. During this entire episode others continuously let me know that another reality was waiting for me outside the hospital. I underwent a complicated operation, recovered slowly and went back to work.

So, I lived in different realities, which were both fragile and contradictory. I received bad and good news. My 'healthy' state after a treatment could turn into disease and sickness in the blink of an eye. I had to cope with uncertainty and distrust in my body. But I also had been exhorted 'to trust myself'. I had to both surrender and to resist. I had to make sense of the different medical stories about my disease. I lived different lives that came with 'the ontologies of medical practice' (Mol, 2007: 181). The consequences of living such a life reached far beyond the illness *per se*.

Medical anthropology has focused on such different realities in the context of the pragmatics of health seeking and 'doing disease'. For example, Mattingly and Hunt (1998) examine 'different forms of rationalities that emerge in everyday efforts to understand and control illness in its real world context' (p. 268). The authors see the different rationalities as having complementary aspects. Within biomedicine there exist multiple realities as well. Hunt and Mattingly argue that formal models of biomedicine constantly shift and are modified in order to 'fit' the 'real world of physical, phenomenological and social lives' (p. 270). The authors focus on 'rationalities', perspectives or modes of thought as frameworks to give meaning and to act.

The argument of multiple realities in biomedicine is developed differently by Annemarie Mol in *The body multiple: Ontology in medical practice* (2007). She studies the 'ways in which medicine attunes to, interacts with, and shapes its objects in its various and varied practices' (p. vii). Her book is not about the different perspectives on the sick body, but on how these perspectives are arrived at or constructed. The author speaks about 'doing disease'. From the interviews and conversations she held in a Dutch hospital, she concluded that 'the humane does not reside exclusively in psychosocial matters' (p. 27) but in the fleshy reality of everyday. Events are made, it is 'ontology in practice', resulting in a body that is present in overlapping realities. A medical condition (in her case atherosclerosis) appears to be many things from one moment, place, apparatus, specialty or treatment to the other. According to Mol this is not fragmentation, but a tactic to make the disease coherent.

A different approach to multiple realities is presented in *Multiple medical realities* (Johannessen and Lazar, 2005). The authors have brought together papers that convey plurality in medicine and related medical pluralism to body and self. They argue that the individual creation of meaning 'in the midst of chaotic life events' is a common theme in understanding both the body and self, as well as medical pluralism. The concept of multiple medical realities does not mean the co-existence of various healing systems, which are more or less separate and independent and from which patients can rationally make a choice. It means fluid and flexible networks based on selective and affinitive organising principles (cf. Burke, 2007).

It is not my intention to give an exhaustive overview of what is written on multiple realities. This is just to briefly outline – in general, and more structured – parts of what I experienced during the course of my illness. Cancer is usually an overwhelming medical experience; it absorbs the energy and time of everyone involved. Stories of cancer patients tell about the desperate attempts to find a cure or relief. They undergo 'dangerous' or invasive treatments; they 'fight' the consequences of such treatments; they look for information about their disease, alternative or complementary treatments; they are confronted with different explanations; they move between bad and good news. A quick scan on internet shows that there are many cancer support groups, cancer centres, chat rooms or web logs worldwide. Many of these groups became popular because they serve an otherwise unmet need: mutual aid and psychosocial needs (Cella & Jellen, 1993). Others focus on education, uncover misconceptions and myths about cancer, or discuss treatments and new possibilities of treatment. Reading through web logs and chat rooms of cancer patients and listening to patients in the cancer clinic, I started to ask myself: Is this really about disease? Or is it perhaps something else, something hidden behind the therapies?

Many of the stories can be categorised as 'this is what happened to me' and often are a way of encouraging others. They are stories of hope. Some have used their cancer experience to develop a broader discussion about sickness. Sontag's *Illness as metaphor* (1978), Frank's *At the will of the body* (1991) and Stoller's *Stranger in the village of the sick* (2004) come to mind. Sontag uses cancer for a critical analysis of the stigmatising effects of cancer metaphors and social categorisation of illness. Frank draws on his experiences to suggest to others that they can make sense of their illness. Stoller uses his experiences of cancer to suggest practical ways to improve quality of life. These works narrate other issues than medical ones that matter to the authors. However, I got the idea that the stories implied a 'happy end' with a significant discovery or lesson; narrators are healed (though sometimes not cured) and the authors claim to be better off at the end. The authors tell their stories when they are physically and emotionally well enough to do so, often after a successful treatment and being recovered enough to write a coherent story. Although authors may have died or experience remissions, there is always some enhancement of health, well-being or vitality in their stories (cf. Thomas Couser, 1997). This is not to say that there is victory or a change in the world. Cancer patients are no heroes. They are 'anti-heroes', raising questions to which there is perhaps no answer, but will have to be asked (Kleinman 2006).

## The 'Jobs' in the cancer clinic: Saving one's soul and integrity

When I could stumble from my hospital bed to the shower, I would wrap myself in a kikoy[2] and cross the corridor to say good morning to a man and a woman who suffered from a similar cancer. The nights often were long, the lights in the corridor sometimes kept us from sleeping, the footsteps of the nurse made us aware that we had constant care, there was snoring, coughing, restless turning, silent crying, and sometimes there was the terrible noise of an emergency when someone got a serious bleeding or became very sick. We had time enough to think, to reflect, and this carried us through the night. During the day we were engaged in examinations, controls, visiting hours, and other activities of the sick. No wonder, our morning talks were not about illness, actions or treatments. Patients find themselves in the situation of Job, the figure in the Old Testament who was seriously challenged by misfortune and nevertheless tried to save his soul.

Mrs Job said: 'I do not speak with my children about this terrible illness. I don't want them to be worried, they are still young.' I said: 'But they see you here, very ill and sad?' She: 'Yes, but during the visits I try to be more or less normal, you know. To be a mother, to show affection and interest in their daily life. You know, it is so frustrating to feel yourself so indifferent to other people sometimes.' Mr. Job: 'You know what is sad? I have lost so many friends. This disease makes you lonely, it can make you bitter. But I cannot be a good companion now. Last night I had a terrible bleeding in my stomach and they brought me to the main medical centre in an ambulance. Even when I feel anger and sometimes – forgive me – hate, I wouldn't wish what happened to me on my worst enemy. But this loss of friends made me worry about my own feelings of friendship.' The struggles and dramas of keeping one's integrity or being a moral person (Kleinman, 2006) began to unfold in the early morning under the clattering of the breakfast car.

Integrity is a concept used in nursing. Usually it is described in terms of keeping up the self-respect, dignity and confidence of the patient (cf. Widäng & Fridlund, 2003). Integrity, a state of being undivided and coherent, is constantly under threat for cancer patients. However, I consider integrity as also having a social dimension, related to the 'soul', a sort of social skin, the boundary between the 'self' and the person.[3]

I had to struggle with questions relating to my commitments to my family and others, to my work. Could I sustain my integrity, a state of being that conflicted so sharply with my situation during the time of several operations, radiation and chemo therapy? I found myself trapped in a gap between my principles and my actions. When everything went well enough I could promise to give a guest lecture in my own university teaching module on theory and practice of medical anthropology, though after some time I had to withdraw. I could plan a trip with my husband, but I had to cancel. 'To be clean'[4] is more complex than to have an active tumour. You believe that moral and social obligations have to be fulfilled. Others expect you to do so too. The side-effects of chemo and radiation fade, you feel appetite again, you force the cancer into the background, but it is still there. People tell you that you look good. Your life has to be seen to be coherent again, but it is not, because of the unpredictability of the disease, a core characteristic of cancer. Increasingly, I became aware of a split between how I felt and how I behaved. I deceived myself and others, and I experienced sometimes that when I told the truth I did not tell it for the sake of truth, but for my own sake. I wondered how much of a burden I could be when I saw the devastating effects of my illness in my husband's and children's faces. I had feelings of guilt, anger and irritation. I realised how difficult it is to remain a moral and social person.

Despite the disease, I felt I had to stand by my family, to be with my friends, and with the PhD students. Or that I had to recover because of a professorship that would enable me to work for human rights, justice and well-being of refugees, something that appealed to my moral principles. Professional success was an important commitment. A conflict between personal and social morality (cf. McFall, 1987) developed. I was a Mrs. Job, who became doubtful about moral values, about others' and my own intentions. The art of being a person of integrity is to remain a social person, to trust and accept that everyone has her own way of 'doing a disease'. I wrote to a friend about Japin's book *De overgave* (*The Surrender*) and cited the main character's words about telling stories: 'No matter how many times you burden people with the story of your past, it does not lighten the burden on your own shoulders. You may tell your entire history, so that they, when they leave, carry this story forever with them. But that is all they carry. A story has no weight. You can talk about your life as often you want, it does not become lighter.'[5] My colleague said that if this were the case, if I seriously believed that, we as anthropologists or professionals who worked in health care might as well stop with our work. There would be no ground for communication. Perhaps she was right, but at that time I had my doubt about a core human activity, perhaps in particular in anthropology: storytelling. I wondered if my work with psychiatric patients and older persons in South Africa, in which the focus was on story-telling, had made a difference. Not that this rather cynical consideration was a new one in anthropology, but this time my wondering was more doubtful. Did story telling really make a difference? And if it did, was my citation of Japin not a mistrust in others who wanted to listen to my story?

## Dealing with fragility

In the beginning we got an almost biblical message from the oncologist: 'Go out and enjoy yourselves …' This message did not fall on deaf ears. We discovered we could still enjoy many things. Such advice is much heard in cases of cancer; it is also much practiced. I heard and read many stories of my fellow-patients who told of how they went on vacation, how they enjoyed a good wine or a book; how they surrounded themselves with beautiful things. People do common things they always do in daily life to keep a sense of continuity. In the cancer clinic 'enjoyment' spatially expresses itself in the front of the building. The restaurant always was full and if you did not know better, it could be a place in the centre of the city, where people came to take a break, to talk, and to drink coffee. Taxi drivers came in and out, looking for their customers. At the front door patients and personnel smoked their cigarettes and talked. Right behind the entrance to the out-patient clinic there was a shop with scarves, wigs, books and shawls, all nicely displayed. Colourful paintings of local artists hung on the walls. People were nicely dressed and laughed or smiled. Sometimes it was as crowded as a shopping centre on a Saturday afternoon. But the careful observer also saw people silently disappearing as fast as they could. This meant: not good news. In our culture, one is hardly allowed to express sadness in the public domain.

As for me, cancer led me back into my life, and into personal reflection. I struggled to remain in the 'normal' daily routine. I answered my emails, read many books, tried to work on some papers, made some paintings and took short walks and canoe trips with my husband. These things helped us to live with the chaos of all the 'realities' we had to deal with.

We developed two projects that absorbed our energy and appealed to our feelings of responsibility. At that time these projects seemed the only way of continuing to be involved in the broader world. The first was a film about swans. The filming and editing hours of shots were a shield against disintegration and fragile realities. But most enjoyable were the encounters with other walkers, older people and people of the village who seemed to enjoy the presence of the swans. We made the film available for children who lived in the nearby village and we used it as an argument for preservation of a fine nature reserve in our district. The other project was the making of a photo book of which the revenues were sent to an South African organisation for young children who had been sexually abused.

I attempted to use my medical anthropological understanding to make sense of what friends and family did – they too were 'doing' my illness – and converted Susan Whyte's argument that it is important to study high-tech techniques in non-Western countries (Whyte, 1997) into a plea for an exploration of non-medical techniques of control, like religious pragmatics or magic such as candle burning in Western countries (Van Dongen, 2008). No doubt, this was more likely an attempt to remain a part of my normal reality – an academic community I believed I belonged to – than to refine a debate. It became clear how important and precious social relationships could be. Being ill is trying to remain a social being, to learn to accept friendship and support, and to remain interested in the lives of others, to maintain sensitivity, integrity and a moral life that is good for the patient and her family. This was difficult enough, especially in times of pain.

## Some final reconsiderations

Many told me to write my story. For a long time, I had a great reluctance to do so. But now I have written a small part of it, leaving out intimacies, doubts, reflections, memories and many other things. Writing is difficult. I cannot concentrate and still wrestle with my doubts. Yet, I also believe that I must write; it is a part of my professional obligation. I cannot claim that my story is about what happens to you when you have cancer. Everybody does her illness in her own way and this may be difficult for others to accept as it is sometimes difficult to accept that everyone has her own unique way of being a patient.

While writing this paper, I received the news that the doctors had found active cancer cells again. Having just returned to work, I will now again have to cancel many appointments with students. Perhaps I will not be able to attend my daughter's final violin recital. At this very moment I am in terrible pain, which unmakes my social world. I have tumbled from the 'village of the healthy' into the 'village of the sick' again. I know what will happen: scans to exclude metastases and to exactly locate the tumor, perhaps radiotherapy in combination with chemo pills and another operation. But I do not belong entirely to the village of the sick; the surgeon said: 'It is remarkable: other than this one place where the cancer is, you are very healthy'. Which is perhaps a scant comfort. But it will help us hold on to the thread of our lives. This is what most cancer patients do.

My experiences have brought about a change in my thoughts about biomedical realities. Anthropological studies of biomedical realities are often patient/family centered and may blur the attempts of doctors, nurses and patients to make medicine a humane matter. But in my experience they do try to understand the other's reality. They do try to help the patients to hold on to the thread of their lives vis-à-vis a fragmenting disease such as cancer. Both patient and health-care professionals suffer and struggle with questions that cannot be answered. When the surgeon told me about the dangers of my third operation, I saw him smile and asked: 'You smile, doctor?' And he answered: 'Yes, but with pain in my heart.' And I believed him. Perhaps anthropology's critique that 'genuine reality is increasingly clouded by professionals whose technical expertise often introduces a superficial and soulless model of the person that denies moral significance' (Kleinman, 2006: 9) is only partly true. It is one (cultural) reality. In particular in cancer, health professionals know that there is more at stake than just a disease. They are moral persons too. They have to bear the sometimes high expectations of patients and often have to admit their powerlessness. Patients and healers are dealing with this chaotic disease and fragile lives in a cultural way, upon which – of course – we should critically reflect. But often doctors try to make their patients' lives as comfortable as possible, much like patients and their family try to do themselves. To elaborate on this issue is outside the scope of this paper. That discussion would be on another level. Within the frame of this paper, I wonder if we should not study 'what is at stake' for both patient and doctor without only focusing on disease and medical realities. We must not overlook that patients and all others, doctors included, have various realities with which they try to deal. Those realities may clash and sometimes contradict each other. In this context, it is perhaps meaningful to share a narrative of a patient I met in a waiting room: "You know, that doctor was at the start of her career. She was busy with machines and my body. It was as if *I* did not exist. I asked her: 'Doctor, can you treat me like a human being?' Cancer tells us about the art of being human and how to learn this art. It tells about social persons who want to save their soul.

I rethink the words in Japin's book about the weight of a story. Often I rethink *Walking stories* (Van Dongen, 2002) in which I described how people suffering with schizophrenia retold and lived their stories in order to do magic, to control their lives, to take care that their illness does not dissolve them as (moral and social) persons. I made a strong claim that stories must be told. But stories often are a burden for patients as well as their caretakers. Yet they hold on. If a story cannot be told, they would pass away, was another claim I made. However, there is also another dimension in storytelling.

The main character also said: 'My memory is like a beehive, you root around in it because you need something sweet, but in the process you disturb the entire breeding place. Suddenly you can't beat off the venom and run for your life' (Japin, 2007: 21). To tell a story may be a painful experience, you do not know what will happen to your words, how they will be explained and interpreted. Some stories simply cannot be told. Because if you do, you lose the connection with others and you will have to choose one reality out of the many realities. Not telling a story can be either silence or denial. Telling a story can be a search for comfort. It can be an attempt to live a moral life. This is not only so for cancer patients, but also for the many displaced persons in the world, for those who suffered violence and grave injustice. This puts a great responsibility on anthropologists (and on doctors and others as well). 'We must attend to consequences rather than convictions', Whyte (1997: 230) argues, '… each term of action has social consequences because it involves assertions of identity, support of other people, and offering of resources.' Stories *can* have a weight for the listener. By way of honest human contact, they connect the souls of tellers and listeners. Stories have a moral weight, because they demand action (cf. Tankink, 2007). But a story alone is not good enough. Perhaps we need an anthropology of sensitivity. I have always wondered how nurses and doctors seem to understand what was going on with a patient without technical devices and without words, simply by using their senses. I also wondered how patients knew before the visit to the doctor what kind of 'news' they would receive. I would like to further explore these phenomena. Often enough deep contact comes without words, or as the result of a joke or a simple wish to have a good weekend. It comes in a smile of recognition in the waiting spaces of the cancer clinics, a hand on your shoulder. And it can come with silence. The surgeon who sits next to your bed and looks at you without words about treatment, progress or medical 'business' can bring more comfort in your fragile world than an assistant who tells in technical terms about the next 'step' of the treatment.

My husband and I could be silent for hours in the hospital. What could we say? It was not necessary to talk. A nurse, who closely observed me, because she thought I may become depressed, told us that she found this very moving. I think of a simple poem of a Dutch poet. Is this a way we could try to grasp the many realities of suffering people? Trying to find words for silence?

## Visit to a patient

My father was silent for a long hour at my bed
When he had put on his hat
I said, well, this conversation
will be easy to resume
No, he said, no, not at all
You'll know if you try it sometime[6]

## Notes

1   The famous North American cyclist, who was cured from cancer and won the Tour de France several times.

2   A colourful cloth that Kenian men and women wear.

3   Hacking (1995: 6) describes the soul as standing for a mix of many aspects of a person. One person speaks with many tongues. The body is the best picture of the soul.

4   Expression used to tell a patient that the cancer cells have disappeared, or are not active anymore.

5   Je kunt nog zo veel mensen met je verleden belasten, het drukt er niet minder om op je eigen schouders. Je kunt ze je hele geschiedenis vertellen, zodat ze wanneer ze vertrekken jouw verhaal voor altijd met zich meedragen. Maar dat is dan ook alles

wat ze dragen. Een verhaal weegt niks. Je kunt over je leven vertellen zo vaak je wilt, lichter wordt het er niet van." (Japin 2007; my translation).

6    Ziekenbezoek

Mijn vader had een lang uur zitten zwijgen bij mijn bed

Toen hij zijn hoed had opgezet

Zei ik, nou, dit gesprek

Is makkelijk te resumeren

Nee, zei hij, nee, toch niet

Je moet het maar eens proberen (Judith Herzberg)

## Bibliography

Burke, Nancy (2007). Book review, *American Anthropologist* 109 (3): 545-546.

Cella, David and S. Yellen (1993). Cancer support groups: the state of the art. Cancer practice 1/1: 56-61.

Couser, Thomas (1997). *Recovering bodies. Illness, disabilities and life writing.* Madison: The University of Wisconsin Press.

Frank, Arthur (1991). *At the will of the body.* Boston: Houghton Mifflin.

Hacking, Ian (1995). *Rewriting the soul. Multiple personality and the sciences of memory.* Princeton: Princeton University Press.

Hunt, Linda (1998). Moral reasoning and the meaning of cancer: Causal explanations of oncologists and patients in Southern Mexico. *Medical Anthropology Quarterly* 12 (3): 298-318.

Hunt, Linda and Cheryl Mattingly (1998). Diverse rationalities and multiple realities in illness and healing. *Medical Anthropology Quarterly* 12 (3): 267-272.

Japin, Arthur (2007). *De overgave.* Amsterdam: Arbeiderspers.

Johannessen, Helle and Imre Lazar (eds.). (2005). *Multiple medical realities: Patients and healers in biomedical, alternative and traditional medicine.* Oxford: Berghahn Books.

Kleinman, Arthur (2006). *What really matters. Living a moral life amidst uncertainty and danger.* Oxford: Oxford University Press.

McFall, Lynne (1987). Integrity. *Ethics* 98 (1): 5-20.

Mol, Annemarie (2007). *The body multiple: Ontology in medical practice.* Durham: Duke University Press.

Scarry, Elaine (1985). *The body in pain. The making and unmaking of the world.* Oxford: Oxford University Press.

Sontag, Susan (1978). *Illness as a metaphor.* New York: Farrar, Strauss and Giroux.

Stoller, Paul (2004). *Stranger in the village of the sick.* Boston: Beacon Press.

Tankink, Marian (2007). My mind as transitional space. Intersubjectivity in the process of analyzing emotionally disturbing data. *Medische Antropologie* 19 (1).

Van Dongen, Els (2002). *Walking stories. An oddnography of what crazy people do with culture*, Amsterdam: Rozenberg Publishers.

Van Dongen, Els (2008). Keeping the feet of the gods and the saints warm: Mundane pragmatics in times of suffering and uncertainty. *Anthropology & Medicine* 15 (3): 263-269.

Weiss, Meira (1997). Signifying the pandemics: Metaphors of Aids, cancer and heart disease. *Medical Anthropology Quarterly* 11 (4): 45-476.

Whyte, Susan R. (1997). Questioning misfortune. The pragmatics of uncertainty in eastern Uganda. Cambridge: Cambridge University Press.

Widäng, Ingrid and Bengt Fridlund (2003). Self-respect, dignity and confidence: Conceptions of integrity among male patients. *Journal of Advanced Nursing* 42 (1): 47-56.

# About the authors

**Rikke Sand Andersen** is an anthropologist and PhD-fellow at the Research Unit for General Practice, Institute of Public Health, University of Aarhus. The main focus of her research is 'patient delay' and how anthropological perspectives may contribute to the understanding of delayed care seeking. She has published in interdisciplinary and medical journals like *BMC Medical Education* and *Migration Letters*. She has recently published an article on methodological problems related to patient delay in *BMC Health Services Research*, and an article on symptom interpretation and 'patient delay' in *Social Science & Medicine* (forthcoming).
E-mail address: rsa@alm.au.dk

**Mabel Gracia Arnaiz** is Professor of Social Anthropology in the University Rovira in Virgili (Tarragona), and researcher in the Observatory of Food (University of Barcelona). She has been visiting researcher at the Centre d'Études de Sociologie, Anthropologie e Histoire (CNRS-EHESS, Paris), at the Centro de Investigaciones y Estudios Superiores en Antropología Social (CIESAS, Mexico D.F) and at the Centre d'Etude du Tourisme et des Industries de l'Accueil (Université de Toulouse Le Mirail 2, Toulouse). She has written diverse articles and books related to the sociocultural study of food, health and genre. Among these publications are, for example, *Paradojas de la alimentación contemporánea* (1996, Icaria, Barcelona), *La transformación de la cultura alimentaria. Cambios y permanencias en un contexto urbano* (1997, Ministerio de Cultura, Madrid), *Somos lo que comemos. Estudios de alimentación y cultura en España* (2002, Ariel, Barcelona), *La alimentación y sus circunstancias: placer, conveniencia y salud* (2004, Odela, Barcelona), *Alimentación y Cultura. Perspectivas antropológicas (*2005, Ariel, Barcelona*) y Comemos como vivimos. Alimentación, salud y estilos de vida* (2006, Odela, Barcelona), and *No Comerás. Narrativas sobre cuerpo, comida y género en el Nuevo milenio* (2007).
E-mail address: mabel.gracia@urv.cat

**Caterina Masana Bofarull** is a social and cultural anthropology graduate and has recently completed her Master's degree in Medical Anthropology and International Health at the Universitat Rovira in Virgili (Tarragona, Spain), where she is currently a PhD student in medical anthropology. She works as a doctoral research fellow in the Department of Anthropology, Philosophy and Social Work at the same university, and also collaborates

in teaching tasks in anthropology subjects. Her dissertation research – supported by the Commission for Universities and Research of the Department of Innovation, Universities and Enterprise of the *Generalitat de Catalunya*, and by the European Social Fund – focuses on the care needs of adults with chronic diseases, with disability and/or dependency, within the context of their family and social network of caregivers. She has participated in several medical anthropology conferences presenting articles related to her research work. Some of this work is scheduled for publication in the coming year.
E-mail address: caterina.masana@urv.cat

**Josep M. Comelles** (1949), MSc and PhD Medicine (UB), PhD Anthropology (EHESS; Paris), MA Psychology (Psicologia, UB), Psychiatrist. Fields of Research: Medical Anthropology, History of Science, Science Studies. Areas: Europe. His main interests are: migration and health, cultural psychiatry, and public policies. Posts: Professor (University Rovira, in Virgili, Tarragona, Spain); visiting Profesor: CIESAS, Mexico; Université Paris X, Nanterre; Université Lumière-Lyon. Author of several books and articles, e.g. *La razón y la sinrazón. Asistencia psiquiátrica y desarrollo del Estado en la España Contemporánea*. Barcelona: PPU (1988), and *Stultifera Navis. La Locura, el poder y la ciudad*. Lleida: Milenio (2006); "Psychiatric Care in relation to the development of the contemporary state: The case of Catalonia", *Culture, Medicine and Psychiatry* 15(2): 193-217, (1991), "The Role of Local Knowledge in Medical Practice: A Trans-Historical Perspective", *Culture, Medicine and Psychiatry* 24: 41-75 (2000). "Writing at the margin of the margin: medical anthropology in Southern Europe", *Anthropology & Medicine* 9(1): 7-23 (2002).
E-mail address: josepmcomelles@gmail.com

**Els van Dongen** (†2009), studied cultural anthropology at the University of Utrecht, where she obtained her Master's degree and a PhD (1994). She held positions at the University of Utrecht, Emerson College, Boston (European centre), and joined the Medical Anthropology Unit at the University of Amsterdam in 1996. She was co-founder of the European network Medical Anthropology at Home. Her research was in the field of (mental) health, immigrants, refugees and elderly. She worked in Europe and South Africa. Her main interests were social memory, trauma and violence (Africa), and immigrants, health and exclusion (Europe). She published widely on mental health, elderly, chronic illness, violence, immigrants and memory. She also worked as a painter, photographer and documentary filmmaker.

**Sylvie Fainzang**, PhD, obtained a HDR (Habilitation à diriger des recherches) at the EHESS (Ecole des Hautes Etudes en Sciences sociales) in Paris in 1997. She is Director of research in the Inserm (Institut national de la santé et de la recherche médicale), and a member of the Cermes (Centre de recherche Médecine, Sciences, Santé & Société). Her main publications are: *Of Malady and Misery. An Africanist Perspective of Illness in Europe* (2000); *Ethnologie des anciens alcooliques. La liberté ou la mort* (1996); *Médicaments et société. Le patient, le médecin et l'ordonnance* (2001); *La relation médecins-malades: information et mensonge* (2006).
E-mail address: sylvie.fainzang@orange.fr
Personal website: http://perso.orange.fr/sylvie.fainzang/

**Rose-Anna Foley** is a PhD student of anthropology at the Institute of Social Sciences, University of Lausanne and research assistant at the School of Health Sciences (HECVSanté), Lausanne. She is also a researcher at the Palliative Care Service, Centre Hospitalier Universitaire Vaudois (CHUV), Lausanne.
E-mail address: rose-anna.foley@unil.ch

**Sylvie Fortin** is Associate Professor at the Department of Anthropology, Université de Montréal. Her current research centers on paediatric hospital practices in the context of urban diversity and how highly specialized and technologically invested environments such as critical care, oncology or neonatal care are sites of negotiation of multiple knowledge, norms, and values amongst health care workers and with families. More broadly, her work centers on social, cultural and religious pluralism and health issues. Migration paths, sociability and identity dynamics in local urban settings as well as in places of origin are also an area of study, with a special interest in North Africa.
E-mail address: sylvie.fortin@umontreal.ca

**Sjaak van der Geest** is Emeritus Professor of Medical Anthropology at the Sociology and Anthropology Department of the University of Amsterdam. He conducted fieldwork in Ghana and Cameroon and published books and articles on various topics in medical anthropology, in particular the cultural context of Western pharmaceuticals in non-Western communities, hospital ethnography, perceptions of sanitation and waste management, and social and cultural meanings of old age in Ghana. Recently published books from his hand are *Social lives of medicines* (Cambridge University Press, 2002;

co-authored with S.R. Whyte and A. Hardon), *Ethnocentrism: Reflections on medical anthropology* (Aksant, 2002, co-edited with R. Reis), and *Generations in Africa: Connections and conflicts*. (2008, Münster: Lit-Verlag, co-edited with Ermute Alber and Susan R. Whyte).
Personal website: www.sjaakvandergeest.nl

**Hans Einar Hem**
Hans Einar Hem gained his degree in Anthropology from the University of Bergen. He is Associate Professor in Health Promotion at Vestfold University College in Norway. He has done fieldwork and local development work in Sudan, Tanzania, Malawi, India, and Sri Lanka, and for shorter periods of time has done fieldwork in several countries, e.g. South Asia, the Balkans and the Middle East. Over the last 15 years he has taught at Vestfold University College and has been instrumental in building up an institute and a Master's programme in Health Promotion.
E-mail address: hehem@mac.com

**Arne T. Høstmark** (1939), Professor emeritus. Until October 2009: (1) Professor of Preventive Medicine (UiO) and Head of Laboratory Group for Health and Environmental Research, Institute of General Practice and Community Medicine; and (2) Professor of Endocrinology at the Norwegian School of Sport Sciences, Oslo. Now retired, but still active in research, Høstmark has been teaching preventive medicine, exercise physiology, biochemistry, endocrinology, nutrition, environmental hygiene etc., has supervised 20 completed PhD candidates and numerous master students, has approximately 150 scientific publications from experimental and epidemiological studies within, for example, carbohydrate and lipid metabolism, physical activity, nutrition, regulation of plasma lipoproteins, cardiovascular risk factors, Type 2 diabetes, post meal blood glucose regulation, diabetes, and acupuncture.
E-mail address: a.t.hostmark@medisin.uio.no

**Helle Johannessen**, Anthropologist, MSc, PhD, is a Professor at the Institute of Public Health, University of Southern Denmark. In fieldwork since the late 1980s she has explored medical pluralism in Denmark, Canada and Italy. Her primary focus has been on the way illness, disease and healing are framed in multiple forms of clinical practice and in political structures. Since 2005 she has been head of a multidisciplinary research unit that uses qualitative methods in the exploration of health-related issues at the

Faculty of Health Sciences, University of Southern Denmark. Further she has received substantial research funding for multidisciplinary research, investigating how qualitative and quantitative methods may supplement each other in research on the effects of treatments.
E-mail address: hjohannessen@health.sdu.dk

**François Kaech** is a PhD student of anthropology and teaching assistant at the Institute of Social Sciences, University of Lausanne. Researcher for Public Health research on the role of resource nurses in elderly homes, in collaboration with the Palliative Care Service, Centre Hospitalier Universitaire Vaudois (CHUV), Lausanne.
E-mail address: Francois.Kaech@unil.ch

**Arantza Meñaca** received a PhD in medical anthropology from the University of Rovira in Virgili (Spain). Her PhD thesis explored the health conditions and health-seeking behaviour of Ecuadorian migrant families in both Spain and Ecuador. She has published several articles related to migration and health, and has presented her findings at various international conferences. Since her PhD she has been working in the international health field in a number of African countries. She is currently a post-doctoral fellow at the Barcelona Centre for International Health Research (CRESIB), where she continues to develop her interests in transnational and international health.
E-mail address: arantzamenaca@aibr.org

**Anne-Lise Middelthon** is a social anthropologist (dr. philos). She is Associate Professor and head of the Section for Medical Anthropology and Medical History, at the Institute of General Practice and Community Medicine, Faculty of Medicine, University of Oslo. While the main focus of her research is on the ongoing medicalisation or pharmacologisation of food in the context of everyday life, the social and cultural dimensions of HIV/Aids has also been a long-term research interest. Semiotics in the tradition of Charles Sanders Peirce constitute a major theoretical framework in her research.
E-mail address: a.l.o.middelthon@medisin.uio.no

**Kåre Moen** is a Medical Doctor and holds a Master's Degree in Public Health. He is currently a Research Fellow at the Section for Medical Anthropology and Medical History at the University of Oslo, working on a

PhD project on HIV and same-sex practicing men in Tanzania. He has previously worked as a general practitioner in Norway, and as an international public health consultant focusing on community health, HIV/AIDS and health impact assessments of large-scale infrastructure development. He has published several books, including a regularly updated comprehensive clinical reference handbook for primary health care physicians (with a parallel edition for non-physicians) and a book on travel medicine. He helped establish and develop *Lommelegen.no*, Norway's most visited consumer-oriented health website.

E-mail address: kare.moen@medisin.uio.no

**Yannis Papadaniel** is a PhD student of anthropology at the Institute of Social Sciences, University of Lausanne; *Diplôme d'études approfondies (DEA)* in anthropology, and teaching assistant at the Institute of Social Sciences, University of Lausanne.

E-mail address: Yannis.Papadaniel@unil.ch

**Mette Bech Risør**, MA, PhD, is a senior researcher at the Research Clinic for Functional Disorders and Psychosomatics, Aarhus University Hospital, Denmark. Risør has a long and in-depth experience with research and teaching in the field of medical anthropology abroad, as well as in Denmark. She has extended network relations to, and knowledge of, other professional milieus, especially health professional, and has profound experience and commitment to working in and with interdisciplinary settings. Her main areas of research interest are illness experience, illness behaviour, health promotion, health systems and knowledge/reasoning – with a theoretical approach from pragmatism, phenomenology and social constructivism.

E-mail address: mettriso@rm.dk

**Ilario Rossi** is Associate Professor at the Institute of Social Sciences, University of Lausanne; and anthropologist at the Polyclinique Médicale Universitaire (PMU), Lausanne. He is author of *Corps et chamanisme. Essai sur le pluralisme médical*, Paris: Armand Colin, 1997, and Rossi I. (eds.), *Prévoir et prédire la maladie: de la divination au pronostic*, Montreuil: Aux lieux d'être, 2007.

E-mail address: Ilario.Rossi@unil.ch